SMOKING:

201 REASONS TO QUIT

SMOKING:
201 REASONS TO QUIT

Muriel L. Crawford

Foreword by
Jack Klugman
Star of stage, screen, and television;
former smoker and cancer survivor;
and anti-smoking activist

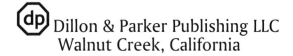 Dillon & Parker Publishing LLC
Walnut Creek, California

Smoking: 201 Reasons to Quit
By Muriel L. Crawford

Published by: **dp** **Dillon & Parker Publishing LLC**
P.O. Box 504
Walnut Creek, California 94597-0504
Website: **www.ReasonsToQuitSmoking.com**
E-mail: **smokingbook@dillon-parkerpublishing.com**

ISBN: 978-0-9819590-0-9
Library of Congress Control Number: 2009902927

First edition
Printed in the United States of America
10 9 8 7 6 5 4 3 2 1

DISCLAIMER
This book is designed to provide information about the hazards of tobacco use. It is sold with the understanding that the publisher and author are not engaged in rendering medical, legal, or any other professional services. If such are required, the services of a competent professional should be sought. This book contains information that is current only up to the printing date. The purpose of this book is to educate. The publisher and author shall have neither liability nor responsibility to any person or entity with respect to any loss or damage caused, or alleged to have been caused, directly or indirectly, by the information contained in this book. If you do not wish to be bound by the above, you may return this book to the publisher for a full refund.

Smoking is a custom loathsome to the eye, hatefull to the nose,
harmfull to the brain, dangerous to the lungs,
and in the black stinking fume therof neerest resembling
the horrible Stigian smoke of the pit that is bottomless.

King James I of England (1604)

TABLE OF CONTENTS

ECONOMIC COSTS–279

HELPING OTHERS QUIT TOBACCO–308

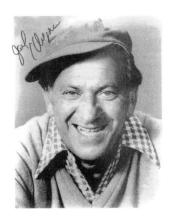

FOREWORD
by
Jack Klugman

I started smoking because I saw John Garfield smoke in the movies. He was my idol, so I smoked like him. I held the cigarette the way he did, took drags on it like he did, threw it away like he did. I smoked heavily for forty years.

In 1970, my smoking almost resulted in my not acting the part of Oscar Madison in the television series *The Odd Couple*. I was sitting in a parked limousine with Tony Randall, who was to play the part of Felix Unger, when suddenly Tony jumped out of the car saying that he couldn't sit in a limousine with me because I was smoking. "I quit!" he said. I bolted from the other side, yelling that Tony was a "finicky pain in the ass" to complain about my smoking. "*I* quit the show," I said. Luckily, the cooler head of Executive Producer Gary Morton prevailed and two limousines were hired, one smoking, one nonsmoking, so neither of us quit.

As I said in my book, *Tony and Me,* in time, Tony became my dearest friend. But he didn't allow smoking on the set of

The Odd Couple. He was fanatically antismoking. He tried many times to get me to quit, because he was worried about what it would do to me. But I never listened. Of course, I wish I had.

In 1974, I kept getting laryngitis, so eventually I went to see a doctor. He told me that I had leukoplakia on my vocal cords. Leukoplakia is a precancerous condition. He said that if I quit smoking the leukoplakia would probably go away, but that if I didn't quit smoking I would lose my vocal cords and my acting career. I stopped smoking for three months. But the day the doctor told me that the leukoplakia was gone, I left his office and bought a pack of cigarettes.

Then, in 1989, while I was rehearsing for a stage revival of *Twelve Angry Men,* I noticed a crack in my voice. I went to my doctor and he saw something he didn't like on my vocal cords. A biopsy showed that I had invasive throat cancer, no doubt caused by my smoking. I wanted to wait for an operation until after the play was over. But the doctor said that I needed an immediate operation. Without the operation, I would die.

The surgeon was hoping to save my vocal cords, but the cancer had spread too much and my right vocal cord had to be reduced to a stump. This meant my speech could never be completely normal, because you need two vocal cords. The cords need to touch each other to produce speech. I could only whisper. I felt that my acting career was over. Instead of *Twelve Angry Men* there was one angry man—me.

But I was lucky. I was cancer-free. In the hospital, Tony Randall was the first friend to visit me. He said that he would find a venue for me if I ever felt like acting again. The support of other cancer survivors was also a wonderful help.

And Gary Catona, a voice-builder, contacted me and said he thought he could help me. I was doubtful, but the strange, almost violent, voice exercises he gave me did help. In time, those voice exercises strengthened my left vocal cord enough so that it could touch the stump of the right cord. People sometimes think that it's uncomfortable for me to talk, but it's just the other way around. The more I talk, the stronger my voice gets.

In 1991, I went back on stage for the first time since my operation. Tony had convinced me to do a benefit stage performance of *The Odd Couple* for the National Actors Theater. Even though I was miked, I was terrified that the audience couldn't hear me. But they laughed at my lines and gradually I relaxed. Now I work on the stage and screen, and travel the world as a spokesman for the American Cancer Society.

I was lucky, but *you* might not be if you smoke. Lots of people, over 400,000 a year in this country, die from smoking. And many more are disabled in one way or another. It took cancer and the loss of my normal speech to motivate me to quit smoking. Don't you wait until something drastic happens before you become motivated. Muriel Crawford has written this book to motivate people to quit smoking before they end up with terrible health problems. Read it carefully—and quit smoking!

Jack Klugman

INTRODUCTION

Many people have an erroneous idea of risk. They may think that driving a car is safer than flying in a commercial airliner, when actually, based upon miles traveled, driving is many times more dangerous than flying—for example, it is far more dangerous to drive 1,000 miles than to fly 1,000 miles. Some people think that radiation from cell phones or power lines is more risky than radiation from the sun, when the opposite is true. Some people fear being struck by lightning more than they fear smoking, but their risk of death from lightning is much smaller than their risk of death from smoking. In the United States, the four leading causes of death are heart disease, cancer, stroke, and chronic lung disease. Smoking greatly increases the risk of all four. Yet one study found that most smokers do not believe that their smoking causes an increased risk of heart attack or cancer. And young people often do not appreciate the risk of experimenting with cigarettes. Beginning smokers tend to think they can quit at any time, and then find that they are addicted to nicotine and that quitting is far more difficult than they thought.

We all engage in activities with some inherent risk, such as driving a car or taking oral contraceptives, but the benefits usually outweigh the risks. This cannot be said for smoking. Simply put, there are no benefits from smoking and the risks are enormous. Smoking is harmful to every part of your body. There is no safe amount to smoke, no safe way to smoke, and no safe cigarette. Quitting is the single best way for a smoker to reduce his or her risk of illness, disability, and early death.

You may already know that the younger you are when you begin to smoke, the more years you smoke, and the more cigarettes a day that you smoke all increase your amount of risk. You may also be aware that your amount of risk is influenced by the type of cigarettes you smoke, how deeply you inhale, other substances you may be exposed to that interact with cigarette smoke (such as asbestos), and whether you have certain diseases (such as asthma), or certain inherited genes. But you may not realize how dramatically you can reduce your risk of many diseases when you quit smoking and remain smoke-free.

The most important reason not to use tobacco is the adverse effect that tobacco use has on your health, and the health of those around you. The United Nations World Health Organization says that cigarette smoking is probably the largest single preventable cause of ill health worldwide. Each year, cigarette smoking causes millions of people to die early and disables millions of others. The illness and suffering that cigarette smoking causes range from irritated eyes to the agony of heart disease, cancer, stroke, and emphysema.

This book does not include all of smoking's harmful effects on health. Some harmful effects have not been included because they affect few people, and others because they have not been studied enough to warrant conclusions. Without a doubt, other harmful effects have yet to be discovered. Tens of thousands of studies have explored the effects of smoking on health. Every month, medical journals around the world publish articles describing new findings. Some end with the observation, "here is one more reason not to smoke." So consider this book an *incomplete* accounting of the ways that smoking ruins your health.

While cigarette smoking is the most destructive form of tobacco use, other forms, such as cigar and pipe smoking, tobacco chewing, and snuff dipping, also cause illness and death. Although cigarette smoking is the main focus of this book, I have included material on these other forms of tobacco use where appropriate.

Secondhand smoke is also harmful. Babies, young children, the elderly, and people with illnesses such as heart disease or asthma are especially vulnerable. Moreover, smoking causes many injuries. For example, cigarettes, matches and lighters cause many fires and explosions that result in deaths, suffering, and disfigurement from burns, as well as property damage. Smoking and driving are a bad combination that increases the likelihood of accidents.

Although health is the most important reason not to use tobacco, there are many other reasons as well. Smoking can strain your family relationships and friendships. It can make you less physically appealing. Moreover, smoking is expensive. In addition to the cost of the cigarettes themselves, smokers pay more for medical care, for several types of insurance, and for cleaning and replacing clothing and household furnishings. On average, smokers earn less than non-smokers, are less likely to be hired or promoted, and recoup less from Social Security and Medicare.

Tobacco can addict you very quickly, both physically and psychologically. For this reason, experimenting with tobacco is dangerous. Attempts to stop using tobacco will probably be difficult if you are addicted to nicotine. Nevertheless, millions of people have stopped smoking, and you can, too. A great deal of help is available if you want to quit, and this book will tell you where to look for that help. But the primary purpose of this book is to persuade you to stay away from tobacco if you don't smoke and, if you do smoke, to motivate you to form a strong commitment to quit. The decision to be a nonsmoker will be one of the most important decisions that you ever make.

DISABILITY AND EARLY DEATH

Disability

1 **Smokers suffer more disabilities than non-smokers, and their disabilities occur earlier and last longer.**

You may dread the prospect of a long disability even more than the prospect of an early death. Smokers on average have more years of disability and dependence on others than nonsmokers. What's more, smokers' disabilities are likely to occur earlier in life and to be more severe. One study found that slender nonsmokers who exercised at least two hours a week remained free of even minor disabilities up to seven years longer than people with unhealthy living habits. Researchers in Florida, a state with many older residents, concluded that smokers enter nursing homes earlier and stay there longer than nonsmokers.

Devastating long-term disabilities can result from smoking-related illnesses such as heart disease, stroke, emphysema, cancer, osteoporosis, and macular degeneration. Studies of older adults show that smokers generally have impaired strength, agility, and balance that can lead to disabling falls. Moreover, smoking contributes to hardening of the arteries in the legs, causing weakness and pain in the leg muscles and impairing the ability to walk and climb stairs. The more you smoke, the more likely you are to lose the abilities that enable you to maintain your independence.

5

Early Death

2 **Cigarette smoking increases your risk of early death, but quitting can increase your life expectancy.**

Cigarette smoking is aptly called "slow suicide." Each year, smoking kills about 440,000 Americans, not including nonsmokers killed by secondhand smoke. Worldwide, smoking kills millions yearly. And smoking just a few cigarettes a day increases your risk of early death by 50 percent, according to one study.

Consider these striking statistics:

- Smoking causes more deaths in the United States than alcohol, cocaine, heroin, automobile accidents, guns, poisons, AIDS, homicide, and suicide combined.

- The United Nations World Health Organization estimates that smoking will kill 50 percent of lifelong smokers. Smoking is the leading preventable cause of early death in the industrialized world. Deaths from smoking are increasing dramatically in the developing world, where half of the men smoke.

- Smoking has killed more Americans in *the last three years* than all the wars fought by the United States since 1775. Thus, cigarettes have been rightly termed the "greatest weapons of mass destruction."

- Men who are lifelong smokers shorten their lives by an average of 13.2 years, women by an average of 14.5 years. But the good news is that the younger you are when you quit smoking, the more your life expectancy increases. If you quit at age 50 you can expect to live six years longer than if you had continued smoking.

■ Smoking kills young people, as well as middle-aged and old people. A study conducted by a life insurer showed that smokers in their twenties had higher death rates than nonsmokers in their twenties.

Few smokers live to an advanced age. Indeed, one study showed that, compared to nonsmokers, only one-tenth as many men who smoke 25 cigarettes a day will live to be 90. The message is clear: if you want to live a long time, *don't smoke*.

HAZARDS TO THE BODY
AS A WHOLE

Dangerous Chemicals

3 **Tobacco smoke contains thousands of chemicals, many of which are dangerous.**

About 4,000 chemicals occur in tobacco smoke. Many chemicals occur naturally in tobacco. Then tobacco crops are sprayed with pesticides and herbicides, adding more. During the manufacture of cigarettes, more chemicals are added. Still more chemicals are created when tobacco burns. The Environmental Protection Agency classifies tobacco smoke as a Class A carcinogen—that is, an agent shown to cause cancer in humans. Moreover, tobacco is often contaminated with a variety of molds that can cause infections, as well as cancer.

According to Action on Smoking and Health (ASH), the national legal-action antismoking organization, cigarettes contain a paint stripper, a lighter fuel, the chemical in mothballs, a poison used in gas chambers, and a rocket fuel. Other chemicals in tobacco smoke include a chemical used in cleaning fluids, a preservative of dead bodies, a chemical used to light blow torches, a material used for brake linings, a heating fuel, an insecticide and weed killer, and a poison with vapors that irritate body tissues.

The three most dangerous components of tobacco smoke are nicotine, carbon monoxide, and tar. *Nicotine*, a highly poisonous chemical, acts both as a powerful stimulant and depressant on your nervous system. Nicotine constricts your blood vessels, increases your heart rate, and affects your hormone production, muscle tension, and skin temperature. Moreover, nicotine is addictive, making smoking difficult to quit.

Nicotine interacts with *carbon monoxide,* a toxic gas in tobacco smoke, making your heart work harder and increasing your risk of heart attack. While nicotine constricts your blood vessels and increases your heart rate, carbon monoxide reduces the oxygen available to your heart.

Tar is composed of particles in tobacco smoke that condense to form a brown, sticky, resin-like mass. Tar contains many chemicals that can cause cancer when applied to the skin or breathing apparatus of laboratory animals. It can do the same to your lungs.

Numerous other chemicals in tobacco smoke cause you harm in a variety of ways. Some interfere with the cleansing action of the hairlike *cilia* that line your respiratory tract. Others are irritants, causing coughing and lung deterioration. And, undoubtedly, chemicals in tobacco smoke act on the body in ways that are still unknown.

Immune System Impairment

4 **Smoking impairs your immune system, hampering its ability to fight infections and cancer.**

Your immune system constantly fights off disease. It is made up of a complicated group of organs, nodes, vessels, white blood cells, and blood proteins that work together to destroy harmful bacteria, viruses, fungi, and other organisms that cause infection. The immune system also destroys cancer cells.

If you have a strong immune system, you are less susceptible to disease than someone with an impaired immune system. Smoking impairs your immune system. Chronic exposure to cigarette smoke decreases the number of some types of white blood cells and causes others to respond less energetically to invading organisms and cancer cells. Protecting your immune system is a compelling reason to avoid smoking. Fortunately, when you quit smoking your immune system starts to recover from the damage within 30 days, although complete recovery may take several years.

Antioxidant Vitamin Depletion

5   **Smoking greatly increases the formation of cell-damaging "free radicals." The body uses up its antioxidant vitamins fighting free radicals, thereby depleting smokers' bodies of these important vitamins.**

Vitamins are chemicals essential to the normal functioning of your body. With a few exceptions, your body cannot manufacture vitamins, but must obtain them from food or vitamin supplements. A balanced diet provides the necessary vitamins for many people. Others require vitamin supplements to assure optimal health. Vitamin supplements should be taken only on the advice of a doctor. Among those likely to need vitamin supplements are the elderly, pregnant women, dieters, alcoholics, and smokers.

Smoking greatly increases the formation of "free radicals," byproducts from the body's oxygen processing. Free radicals damage cells and cause the body to degenerate over time. The antioxidant vitamins—vitamin C, beta-carotene and other carotenoids, and vitamin E—can neutralize free radicals, but are used up in the process, thereby depleting smokers' bodies of these vitamins.

High levels of the three antioxidant vitamins in the body may help lower your risk of degenerative diseases—heart disease, cancer, osteoporosis, cataracts, and age-related macular degeneration. But studies show that, on average, smokers have lower blood levels of antioxidant vitamins than nonsmokers—40 percent lower in the case of vitamin C. Vitamin C is a powerful antioxidant that improves wound healing, fights infection, and helps the body absorb iron. It is also necessary to the formation of collagen, a strong, fibrous substance in skin, tendons, ligaments, bone, cartilage, capillaries, and dental tissues.

Vitamin C is found in many orange, green, and red vegetables and fruits. These should be part of your daily diet, since vitamin C can't be stored in your body. Beta-carotene and many other carotenoids are found in highly colored vegetables and fruits such as carrots, squash, sweet potatoes, cantaloupe, broccoli, apricots, and spinach. Vitamin E is found in vegetable seed oils, nuts, legumes, dark green leafy vegetables, wheat germ, and eggs.

A diet that is rich in foods containing antioxidant vitamins is important for everyone, but especially for smokers. Unfortunately, studies of populations in many countries show that smokers generally have poorer diets than nonsmokers. Some physicians advise their patients who smoke to supplement their diets with a multivitamin pill, and/or with vitamins C and E. Beta-carotene supplements usually are not recommended because studies indicate an increased risk of lung cancer for smokers taking these pills.

BLOOD VESSEL DISEASE, HEART DISEASE, AND STROKE

Blood Vessel Disease

6 **Smoking puts you at major risk for athero-sclerosis, a dangerous condition in which plaque deposits form in artery walls.**

The arteries are a system of branching, elastic tubes through which your heart pumps oxygen-filled blood to all parts of your body. *Arteriosclerosis* is a general term for any hardening and loss of elasticity of the arteries. *Atherosclerosis*, a form of arteriosclerosis, results when deposits of plaque form in the walls of arteries. These plaque deposits can narrow the arteries. A plaque deposit also can burst and form a blood clot that blocks an artery. If the artery supplies blood to the heart, a heart attack results. If the artery supplies blood to the brain, a stroke results. Atherosclerosis kills between one-third and one-half of all Americans. It is the most dangerous disease on earth.

Atherosclerosis is a major cause not only of death, but also of crippling disability. It affects arteries all over the body, including those supplying blood to the heart, brain, kidneys, intestines, and other vital organs. It also affects arteries supplying blood to the eyes, arms, and legs. Heart attacks, strokes, kidney disease, blindness, and amputation of limbs are only some of the results of atherosclerosis.

Atherosclerosis is a long-term, progressive disease that usually doesn't produce symptoms until artery blockage is advanced. When symptoms do develop, they are likely to be gradual. You first may experience heart pain (angina) during exercise because plaque buildup in a coronary artery (an artery supplying the heart with blood) prevents adequate oxygen supply to your heart. But even without symptoms, plaque can rupture and cause a heart attack or stroke. In some cases, the first symptom of atherosclerosis is death.

Many scientists think that atherosclerosis starts because high blood pressure, high levels of cholesterol and triglyceride in the blood, or smoking, damage the inside of the arteries. Diabetes, obesity, and lack of exercise are also risk factors for atherosclerosis.

One large study found that atherosclerosis progresses 50 percent faster in smokers than in people who have never smoked. Smoking not only damages the walls of arteries, it also promotes high blood pressure, diabetes, and blood clotting. In addition, smoking lowers high-density cholesterol (HDL), the "good cholesterol" that helps remove excess cholesterol from your blood. But the good news is that quitting smoking tends to raise your HDL.

There is even more good news. Adoption of a healthy lifestyle can reverse atherosclerosis. A healthy lifestyle includes a low-saturated-fat, high-fiber diet; weight control; exercise; stress management; medication if your doctor recommends it; and not smoking. Start now to lead a healthy lifestyle and you will increase your odds of a long life without disability.

7 If you smoke, you have three to four times more risk of developing peripheral artery disease than a nonsmoker has. Peripheral artery disease can result in leg pain, open sores, gangrene, and amputation.

Peripheral artery disease (PAD) occurs when plaque builds up in the aorta, the body's main artery, or in the arteries of the legs or arms—that is, atherosclerosis can cause PAD. Significant plaque buildup in arteries serving the heart and brain often accompanies PAD, increasing the danger of heart attack or stroke.

PAD progresses gradually. Most people with PAD don't have symptoms. In those with symptoms, leg pain is often the first symptom. The leg pain occurs during walking, because the leg muscles need additional oxygen-rich blood then, blood that the clogged arteries can't provide. Later, when the arteries become even more clogged, there may be leg pain even while resting. Chronic poor circulation in the feet and legs can lead to breakdown of the skin and open sores. Gangrene (death of body tissue) develops in severe cases, requiring amputation of the foot or leg.

If you smoke, you have three to four times more risk of developing PAD than a nonsmoker has. If you have already developed PAD, quitting smoking will slow the progression of the disease and reduce the likelihood of amputation. Also, surgery to bypass or unblock the diseased blood vessels is more apt to be successful if you are a nonsmoker.

Smokers with diabetes are especially prone to PAD. The prognosis of PAD in a diabetic smoker is grim because diabetics are more likely to develop foot sores, and their sores are slower to heal and more likely to become infected.

For these reasons and others discussed in this book, if you are a diabetic you are strongly advised not to smoke.

Buerger's disease is a type of PAD that occurs almost exclusively in smokers. Lifetime nonsmokers have almost no risk of Buerger's disease. Most people with Buerger's disease are male cigarette smokers between the ages of 20 and 45. Five percent are female smokers. Buerger's disease is an inflammation of blood vessels in the lower legs, feet, wrists, and hands. The inflammation causes these vessels to narrow, so that the blood supply to the extremities is impaired. Buerger's disease can cause pain, open sores, and gangrene. The fingers, toes, or even the legs, may have to be amputated. Fortunately, Buerger's disease is uncommon.

If a smoker diagnosed with Buerger's disease continues to smoke, the disease will become progressively worse. On the other hand, marked improvement is likely when a smoker quits early in the course of the disease.

8 Smoking is a major risk factor for high blood pressure, the "silent killer."

As blood circulates through your arteries it exerts force, or pressure, against them. Blood flows in spurts created by the pumping of your heart. With each heartbeat, blood is pumped into your arteries, raising the pressure. Between heartbeats, pressure decreases. So, when your blood pressure is measured, it is stated in two numbers (115/70, for example), the higher number representing maximum pressure when your heart beats, and the lower number the pressure between heartbeats. A blood pressure level less than 120/80 is considered normal.

You probably know that physical activity or stress temporarily raises your blood pressure. This is not high blood pressure, or *hypertension*. High blood pressure is a condition in which *consistent, excessive* pressure is exerted against your artery walls. High blood pressure is common. Nearly one-third of American adults have it, and nearly one-third of those who have it don't know that they have it. By itself, high blood pressure causes no symptoms. But, if untreated, it can result in early death from stroke, heart attack, heart failure, or kidney failure. This is why high blood pressure is called the "silent killer." Moreover, evidence is increasing that there is a link between high blood pressure and mental deterioration.

You can help prevent or reduce high blood pressure by

- eating a low-saturated-fat, low-salt, diet containing lots of vegetables, fruits, and whole grains,

- losing weight if you are overweight,

- getting at least 30 minutes of exercise on most days,

- limiting alcohol to two drinks per day if you are a man, and one drink per day if you are a woman,

- and not smoking!

Smoking is a major risk factor for high blood pressure. Nicotine constricts your small blood vessels and temporarily raises your blood pressure. Dr. Rose Marie Robertson, a specialist in cardiovascular diseases and a professor of medicine at Vanderbilt University says, "Absolutely nothing is worse for blood pressure. Every cigarette you smoke raises pressure by five to ten points, and it stays up for as long as ninety minutes." Fortunately, quitting smoking can lower your blood pressure. And there are medications that can lower high blood pressure if quitting smoking and other health measures are not enough to lower it to normal.

9   **Smoking increases your risk of developing Type 2 diabetes and increases the damage that diabetes does to blood vessels.**

Diabetes mellitus is characterized by the body's inability to process blood sugar properly. Diabetes tends to run in families. There are two types of diabetes: Type 1 diabetes—commonly called "juvenile diabetes"—which usually develops before age 30 and requires multiple, daily insulin injections for survival; and Type 2 diabetes, which usually develops after age 30 and may not require insulin injections. Over 90 percent of diabetics have Type 2 diabetes. In the United States, Type 2 diabetes is reaching epidemic proportions as baby-boomers reach middle age, and as the incidence of obesity and inactivity in the population increases.

Controlling diabetes is difficult, but vital. Diabetes can damage blood vessels all over the body. Control of diabetes requires a special diet, weight control, exercise, blood sugar monitoring (usually two or three times a day), and, in many cases, oral medication or insulin injections. The numerous possible complications of diabetes are less likely to occur when diabetes is well controlled. These complications include heart attack, heart failure, stroke, kidney disease, peripheral artery disease, blindness, and nerve damage.

Several studies indicate that you are more likely to develop Type 2 diabetes if you smoke. One study indicates that smokers are almost twice as likely to develop Type 2 diabetes as nonsmokers. If you already have diabetes, it is *vital* that you refrain from smoking. Atherosclerosis (plaque formation in the artery walls) and arteriosclerosis (thickening and loss of elasticity of the artery walls) are much more common in diabetics, appear at a younger age, and advance more rapidly. Diabetes also can damage capillaries, the tiny blood vessels that nourish individual body cells. Smoking increases the risk that this damage will occur. The combination of diabetes and smoking does far more blood vessel damage than the sum of their individual effects.

Most diabetics die of heart disease because of damage to the blood vessels that nourish the heart. Smoking makes this outcome even more likely. Many diabetics, especially Type 1 diabetics, die of kidney disease because of damage to blood vessels in the kidneys. In the United States, diabetes is the most common cause of extreme loss of kidney function (end-stage renal disease). People with end-stage renal disease often undergo years of kidney dialysis, a treatment that can have many complications, including pain. Some undergo kidney transplant. Smoking promotes the progression of kidney disease in diabetics.

Diabetics who smoke have a risk of early death 11 times that of nonsmokers who are not diabetic. Quitting smoking reduces that risk, although the risk from smoking remains high for several years and depends on the number of years that the person smoked. Young diabetics, who usually have a more severe form of the disease, *must not* begin smoking. If you have a close relative who is diabetic you have a higher-than-average risk of developing diabetes and should avoid smoking.

10 If you smoke you are much more likely than a nonsmoker to develop an aneurysm that may rupture and cause death or severe disability.

An *aneurysm* is a bulge in a blood vessel at a weak spot in the vessel wall. Aneurysms can occur anywhere in the body, but most occur in the major artery in the chest and abdomen, called the *aorta,* or in an artery supplying the brain. A rupture in an artery supplying the brain results in a *hemorrhagic stroke.*

Sometimes a weakness in a blood vessel wall is present at birth. This can cause an aneurysm. Trauma or infection cause other aneurysms. But the most common cause of aneurysms is plaque deposits that weaken artery walls—that is, atherosclerosis. Smoking is a major risk factor for atherosclerosis. High blood pressure is also a risk factor for atherosclerosis and, furthermore, puts extra stress on weakened artery walls. Therefore, high blood pressure is a major risk factor for the development and rupture of aneurysms. Smoking constricts blood vessels and makes high blood pressure worse.

Ruptured aortic aneurysms kill at least 9,000 Americans each year, four times as many men as women. A ruptured aortic aneurysm is almost always fatal. Most aortic aneurysms do not cause symptoms until they grow large enough to rupture. Even after symptoms appear, they are easily confused with symptoms of other conditions, so misdiagnosis is common. Once a rupture occurs, there is massive internal bleeding. Many people with a ruptured aortic aneurysm die before reaching the operating room. Even with immediate surgery, a person with a ruptured aortic aneurysm has less than a 50 percent chance of surviving.

The U.S. Preventive Services Task Force recommends that all males between the ages of 65 and 75 who are smokers, or former smokers, undergo an ultrasound test for aortic aneurysm. The Task Force did not recommend screening after age 75 because surgery to repair an aortic aneurysm is riskier at older ages. But other experts think that female smokers, female former smokers between 65 and 75, and anyone over 75 who has ever smoked, should also be tested.

Open chest surgery to repair an aortic aneurysm that has not ruptured has been the conventional treatment. Newer treatment involves placing a tube-shaped graft called a "stent" inside the artery. When used in appropriate cases, stenting has the advantage over open chest surgery of being minimally invasive, quicker, and safer.

Smoking greatly increases your risk of developing an aortic aneurysm. Consider:

- Current smokers are 7.6 times more likely than lifelong nonsmokers to develop an abdominal aortic aneurysm.

- Aortic aneurysms grow more rapidly in smokers than in nonsmokers.

- A smoker's risk of developing an aortic aneurysm declines, although very slowly, when he or she quits smoking.

11 Smoking increases your risk of developing dangerous blood clots in the legs, a condition called "deep vein thrombosis."

As people spend more time sitting in cramped airplane seats, concern has risen about *deep vein thrombosis* (DVT), sometimes called "economy class syndrome." DVT is the formation of a blood clot in a leg. Such a clot may break off and travel to the lungs. A blood clot that travels to the lungs is called a *pulmonary embolism*. A large pulmonary embolism can quickly cause death. A hospital near London's Heathrow Airport reported 30 such deaths within three years.

Like air travel, prolonged car or train travel, long hours sitting at a desk, or illnesses that keep you off your feet can lead to DVT. Smokers are more likely than nonsmokers to be immobilized by heart attack, heart failure, stroke, or chronic obstructive pulmonary disease. And DVT is usually the result of sluggish blood flow because of immobility, *plus* another factor, such as smoking, that increases the tendency of blood to clot. Thus, smoking puts you at increased risk of DVT and pulmonary embolism.

Heart Disease

12 Heart disease is the number one killer of Americans. About 30 percent of heart disease results from smoking.

Heart disease is the number one killer of both men and women in the United States. About 30 percent of heart disease results from smoking. This alone is reason enough for you to quit smoking.

The heart, a muscular pump, supplies your body with oxygen and nutrients by pumping your blood through a 60,000-mile network of arteries, veins, and capillaries. Every cell, every tissue, every organ—including your heart itself—depends on oxygen and nutrients in the blood pumped by your heart.

The nicotine and carbon monoxide in tobacco smoke make your heart work harder. Nicotine makes your heart pump faster and constricts your blood vessels, while carbon monoxide reduces the amount of oxygen in your blood. Moreover, smoking contributes to the loss of elasticity of your artery walls, and to the development of atherosclerosis, in which plaque deposits form in your artery walls. It taxes your heart to pump blood through inelastic, narrow arteries. To make matters worse, smoking increases the incidence of blood clots. If a coronary artery providing blood to the heart muscle becomes blocked by a blood clot, a heart attack results. Thus, smoking increases your risk of heart attack, and of the other manifestations of heart disease, including angina (heart pain), heart failure, cardiac arrest, and heart rhythm disturbances. (These are all discussed below.)

Women who are nonsmokers typically get heart disease much later than men. Not so for women who smoke. One study concluded that, on average, female smokers have heart attacks 14 years earlier than female nonsmokers. Male smokers have heart attacks six years earlier than male nonsmokers. Thus, smoking is more dangerous for women than for men. But quitting cigarettes is highly beneficial for everybody. Your risk factors for developing heart disease decline nearly to those of nonsmokers within two years after you quit.

13 Smoking is a cause of angina, makes angina worse, and reduces the effectiveness of treatment.

Angina pectoris, usually called simply *angina*, is temporary heart pain due to a lack of oxygen to the heart muscle. Angina is a common problem, afflicting six million Americans. Angina results when coronary arteries are narrowed by deposits of plaque—that is, by atherosclerosis.

The two main kinds of angina are unstable angina and stable angina. Unstable angina can occur without physical exertion, as when a person is at rest. It does not follow a pattern, as stable angina does. Unstable angina is an emergency condition, as a heart attack may soon follow.

Stable angina occurs when the heart muscle's demand for oxygen is increased during exercise, at times of emotional stress, during exposure to cold or hot weather, or after a heavy meal. The pain usually starts in the heart, but may spread to the throat, jaw, back, or arms. The afflicted person may sweat, have difficulty breathing, or feel nauseated or dizzy. Symptoms and pain abate when the demand for oxygen is decreased, as after a short rest. Stable angina does not damage the heart muscle as a heart attack can, because with angina the blood flow is reduced, whereas with a heart attack blood flow is cut off suddenly and completely. However, a person with stable angina is at risk of having a heart attack or cardiac arrest. Steps to prevent these include controlling weight, blood pressure and diabetes; lowering LDL (bad) cholesterol; and not smoking.

Smoking is a cause of angina because smoking contributes to the development of atherosclerosis. Moreover, tobacco smoke contains carbon monoxide and nicotine. Carbon monoxide replaces oxygen in the blood and nicotine constricts blood vessels, both of which make angina worse. Angina sufferers who quit smoking often enjoy an immediate reduction in the number of stable angina episodes.

The pain of angina can be relieved by nitroglycerine, a prescription drug that relaxes and opens the arteries. But smoking reduces nitroglycerine's effectiveness because the nicotine in tobacco smoke constricts the arteries.

14 If you smoke you are five times more likely than a nonsmoker to suffer a heart attack in your 30s or 40s, twice as likely as a nonsmoker to die of a first heart attack, and twice as likely to suffer a second heart attack.

A heart attack occurs when an artery that provides blood to the heart becomes blocked and part of the heart muscle dies. Heart attack survivors have a greatly increased risk of suffering another heart attack. Some are permanently disabled because a large area of heart muscle has been destroyed.

Generally speaking, smokers suffer first heart attacks at much younger ages than nonsmokers. If you smoke you are five times more likely than a nonsmoker to have a heart attack in your 30s or 40s. Although heart attacks rarely strike women under age 45, when they do the woman is nearly always a smoker. Furthermore, a smoker is about twice as likely to die from a first heart attack as a nonsmoker, and more likely to die suddenly, within an hour. Smoking after a heart attack doubles your risk of having another heart attack.

Recent studies have found that up to 94 percent of heart attack patients have at least one of four major risk factors:

- Smoking

- High cholesterol

- High blood pressure

- Diabetes

The role that smoking plays in the development of high cholesterol, and how smoking makes high blood pressure worse have already been discussed. Smoking also increases the risk of developing the most common type of diabetes. But even if you have none of the other three risk factors, smoking by itself is a risk factor for heart attack.

15 Smoking is a major risk factor for heart failure, a common and serious medical condition.

Heart failure is the progressive weakening of the heart so that it can no longer pump blood efficiently. Heart failure usually develops slowly as the heart loses its pumping ability. The heart gradually grows larger and beats faster in an attempt to compensate for its decreased ability to pump blood. The body retains salt and water in an attempt to increase blood volume. Eventually, these attempts to compensate are not enough and the symptoms of heart failure appear. These symptoms include fatigue, breathing difficulties, and swollen feet and ankles.

In the United States, there is an epidemic of heart failure. Five million people have this condition. It is diagnosed in 550,000 people each year. Although treatments are improving, many people still die from heart failure. Chronic lung disease, diabetes, heart attack, high blood pressure, or coronary arteries narrowed by atherosclerosis can weaken the heart and result in heart failure. Smoking contributes to all these conditions, and is therefore a major risk factor for heart failure.

A healthy lifestyle is essential for people with heart failure. And early treatment of heart failure can sometimes keep it from worsening, or even reverse its progress. If you have developed heart failure you can improve your chances of living longer by controlling cholesterol, high blood pressure, diabetes, and weight—and by quitting smoking.

16 Smoking doubles your risk of cardiac arrest.

Cardiac arrest is the leading cause of death in men aged 20 to 60. More than 50 percent of deaths from heart disease are due to cardiac arrest. Between 250,000 and 450,000 Americans suffer cardiac arrest yearly. Only about five percent survive. Unlike a heart attack, cardiac arrest strikes suddenly and without warning. The heart quivers (a rhythm disturbance called *ventricular fibrillation*) instead of pumping blood, or suddenly stops beating altogether. The person collapses within seconds, stops breathing, and has no pulse. If normal heart pumping is not restored within a few minutes, death occurs. Unfortunately, most cases of cardiac arrest don't happen where trained medical personnel, and machines called defibrillators, are available to quickly restart the heart. Family members or bystanders can sometimes successfully perform cardiopulmonary resuscitation (CPR) until medical personnel arrive, but someone trained in CPR must begin it quickly—ideally within two minutes of cardiac arrest.

The increasing availability of portable defibrillators in public places such as airplanes, office buildings, stadiums, shopping malls, and in fire and police vehicles, has somewhat improved the outlook for people who suffer cardiac arrest. Sometimes a portable defibrillator is kept in the home of a patient known to be at high risk for cardiac arrest. Or such a patient may have a small defibrillator implanted in his chest. A defibrillator that can be strapped to a patient's chest has recently become available. This defibrillator can be worn 24 hours a day, except when bathing.

Most people who suffer cardiac arrest have atherosclerosis of their coronary arteries and many have already had a heart attack. Clearly, the best way to avoid cardiac arrest is to pursue the healthy lifestyle that helps prevent atherosclerosis and heart attack, including not smoking. Smoking doubles your risk of cardiac arrest.

17 Smoking triggers skipped or rapid heartbeats, and increases your risk of dangerous arrhythmias.

Your heart has a natural pacemaker, the *sinus node*, that controls its rate and rhythm. Your heart rate normally varies with activity, increasing with exertion to supply your body with additional oxygen. Sometimes the normal pacing of the heart is disturbed and the heart rate becomes too fast or too slow. Heart rhythm can also deviate from normal, as when the heart skips a beat. An *arrhythmia* is any deviation from the heart's normal rate or rhythm.

It is normal for the heart to have small disturbances, such as an occasional skipped beat—actually a single premature beat, followed by a pause. This feels like a thumping or fluttering in your chest and may sometimes cause a brief but frightening feeling that your heart has stopped. Menstruation, decongestants, alcohol, caffeine, lack of sleep, anxiety, and nicotine—all can trigger skipped beats. Because of the nicotine in tobacco smoke, and because smokers tend to have more anxiety and insomnia than nonsmokers, smokers are more likely to have skipped beats. If skipped beats occur frequently, or are accompanied by other symptoms, medical attention is needed.

Tachycardia, when the number of heartbeats exceeds 100 per minute, is a natural response to physical exertion and may occur at other times because of anxiety, fever, or dehydration. Tachycardia in a person with a healthy heart usually is not a cause for concern. As with skipped beats, the nicotine in cigarette smoke can trigger tachycardia.

A potentially dangerous arrhythmia called *atrial fibrillation* occurs when the upper chambers of the heart, the *atria,* contract in an uncoordinated, patternless manner. Atrial fibrillation sometimes promotes the formation of a blood clot that can travel to the brain and cause a stroke. Atrial fibrillation commonly occurs in people who have atherosclerosis of the arteries supplying the heart muscle with blood (the coronary arteries). Smoking contributes to the development of atherosclerosis, and therefore to the occurrence of atrial fibrillation.

Ventricular fibrillation, the most dangerous arrhythmia, occurs when the lower chambers of the heart, the *ventricles,* contract so fast that the heart is reduced to a chaotic quiver and cannot pump blood. Ventricular fibrillation is an extreme medical emergency. If the heart is not shocked back into a normal rhythm with a defibrillator, cardiac arrest and death can occur within minutes. The impact of smoking on ventricular fibrillation and cardiac arrest was discussed in more detail in Number 16 above.

18 **Heavy smoking, and heart and lung diseases caused by smoking, can induce a condition called "secondary polycythemia" that decreases the oxygen delivered to body cells and increases the danger of blood clots that can result in heart attack or stroke.**

Your red blood cells contain hemoglobin that binds with oxygen in your lungs. Your blood carries this life-giving oxygen to cells throughout your body. Carbon monoxide—a colorless, odorless gas—has a much greater power than oxygen to bind with hemoglobin. Carbon monoxide therefore displaces oxygen in the red blood cells, depriving your cells of oxygen. Death can occur if a person breathes a large quantity of carbon monoxide—for example, from car exhaust in a closed garage, or from a malfunctioning furnace in a house with the doors and windows closed.

Tobacco smoke also contains carbon monoxide. In smokers, the number of red blood cells carrying carbon monoxide varies with the amount of smoke inhaled. Studies indicate that the number of red blood cells carrying carbon monoxide averages about six percent in moderate smokers and eight percent in heavy smokers, but can be as high as 21 percent. Cigar smokers who inhale tend to have the highest percentage of red blood cells carrying carbon monoxide.

As the carbon monoxide in tobacco smoke occupies more and more red blood cells, the remaining red blood cells hold onto oxygen tightly, making it even more difficult for body cells to get the oxygen they need. In an effort to compensate for this oxygen deprivation, the body produces more red blood cells. This excessive number of red blood cells results in *secondary polycythemia,* a condition often found in people who smoke heavily.

People who have heart disease or a lung disease called *chronic obstructive pulmonary disease* (COPD) also suffer oxygen deficiency because the heart or lungs are not working properly. Again, the body attempts to compensate by increasing the number of red blood cells, which can cause secondary polycythemia. Smoking is a major cause of both heart disease and COPD.

Common symptoms of secondary polycythemia are fatigue, headache, breathlessness, dizziness, and lightheadedness. In secondary polycythemia, blood plasma (the fluid in which blood cells are suspended) may be reduced. The blood, with its reduced plasma and excessive number of red cells, becomes thicker and stickier. This impedes the blood's usually rapid flow and decreases the quantity of oxygen delivered to body cells. Moreover, slow-flowing, thick, sticky blood is more likely than normal blood to form clots that can result in a heart attack, stroke, or other serious health problems.

If you develop secondary polycythemia due to the carbon monoxide in tobacco smoke, you can be cured if you quit smoking. Long-term oxygen therapy reduces excess red blood cells in people with secondary polycythemia due to heart disease or COPD, but only if they quit smoking.

Stroke

19 **In the United States, stroke is the third leading cause of death, but the number one cause of adult disability. *Ischemic stroke* is the most common kind of stroke. Smoking at least doubles your risk of stroke.**

A minority of strokes occur when an artery supplying the brain ruptures (hemorrhagic stroke). But most strokes occur when a blood clot or a fatty deposit blocks an artery supplying the brain with blood (ischemic stroke). Atherosclerosis is a major cause of ischemic stroke. Smoking is a cause of atherosclerosis and makes your blood more likely to clot, and thus more likely to block an artery supplying the brain.

Only heart disease and cancer cause more deaths in this country than strokes. But strokes are the *leading* cause of disability among American adults. The effects of a stroke may be temporary or permanent. These effects may include difficulty with speaking, problems with vision, inability to control emotions, memory loss, paralysis, or coma. Having a stroke can change your life in a matter of moments—causing handicaps that make you dependent on others physically, emotionally, and financially.

When you smoke, you at least double your risk of having a stroke. One study of strokes among smokers finds the risk to be six times greater for smokers than for nonsmokers. And smokers are likely to have strokes at younger ages than nonsmokers. Prevention of stroke is much more effective than treatment.

The good news is that as soon as you quit smoking your risk of stroke begins to decline. Five to 15 years after you quit, your risk of stroke from smoking disappears.

20 High blood pressure, aneurysm, and cancer are the main causes of a dangerous type of stroke, called *hemorrhagic stroke*. Smoking makes high blood pressure worse and greatly increases the risk of aneurysm and cancer.

A rupture in an artery supplying the brain with blood causes a dangerous type of stroke called *hemorrhagic stroke*. Hemorrhagic stroke is more likely to cause death than ischemic stroke. Current smokers are three and one-half times more likely to suffer hemorrhagic stroke than lifetime nonsmokers.

Unlike ischemic stroke, in which blood to part of the brain is cut off, in hemorrhagic stroke the brain is flooded with blood. The blood irritates the brain and causes swelling. Moreover, the blood forms a mass called a hematoma that presses on the brain. Immediate treatment of hemorrhagic stroke is essential.

High blood pressure is one cause of hemorrhagic stroke. High blood pressure stresses the artery walls and may cause them to rupture. Smoking makes high blood pressure worse.

Sometimes a weak spot in an artery supplying the brain with blood (an aneurysm) ruptures and causes a hemorrhagic stroke. The statistics from clinical studies concerning smoking and aneurysms in arteries supplying the brain tell a story similar to that for aortic aneurysms:

- People who smoke heavily have a higher risk of developing an aneurysm in an artery supplying the brain than light smokers.

- The risk of an aneurysm in an artery supplying the brain gradually declines when people stop smoking, but they must abstain from cigarettes for more than ten years for the risk to decline to that of lifetime nonsmokers.

Cancer also can cause bleeding in the brain. This is especially apt to happen when the cancer has spread to the brain from a distant site in the body. For example, lung cancer often spreads to the brain. And most lung cancer is caused by smoking.

CANCER

Causes of Cancer

21 Chemical mutagens in tobacco can damage your genes and cause cancer.

Cells are the basic building blocks of your body. A human body begins as one cell, the fertilized egg. The egg divides into two cells, and those cells divide in a pattern controlled by the genes. The 30,000 genes in each cell contain the blueprint for the entire body. Your genes direct the development and functioning of all your organs and systems.

When a cell divides, each of the two resulting cells receives a copy of all your genes, but sometimes that copy is imperfect. The cell with the imperfect copy will then pass on that imperfection when it divides. This is called *mutation*. Mutation may have only mild effects on the body, or it can be deadly, depending on the gene that was imperfectly copied.

Mutagens are agents that can cause genes to mutate. Mutagens include X-rays, radioactive substances, ultraviolet light, and chemicals in tobacco. A carcinogen is one type of mutagen, the type that causes cancer.

Cancer is uncontrolled cell division. The p53 tumor suppressor gene helps control cell division. Mutation in the p53 gene occurs in almost half of all types of cancer. A mutated p53 gene cannot properly control cell division. Recent studies of cancers indicate that people who use tobacco have twice as many mutations in the p53 gene as people who do not. If tobacco smoke causes the p53 gene in one lung cell to mutate, that cell might begin dividing relentlessly, resulting in a cancerous tumor.

Many other genes also play a role in cell division, and tobacco may cause mutations in these genes as well. The propensity of tobacco to cause mutations in genes helps explain why nearly one-third of all cancers are due to tobacco use.

22 Tobacco use is the major single cause of cancer deaths in the United States.

Cancer is a group of diseases characterized by the uncontrolled division and spread of abnormal cells. After heart disease, cancer is the second greatest killer in the United States, causing nearly one in four deaths. Cancers of the lung, mouth, throat, and larynx are especially likely to develop in smokers.

Although there are numerous direct and indirect causes of cancer—including a poor diet, obesity, heredity, industrial pollutants, radiation, and certain viruses—tobacco use is the major single cause of cancer deaths. The smoke from just a few cigarettes every day increases cancer risk more than anything else you are likely to be exposed to. Cancer deaths in the United States could be reduced by 31 percent over time if all Americans avoided tobacco. The increased danger of heart disease and cancer are the two most important reasons not to use tobacco.

Tobacco smoke contains *carcinogens*, cancer-causing substances that travel through the bloodstream to distant sites in the body. Tobacco that is held in the mouth or chewed (smokeless or spit tobacco) also contains carcinogens that can cause mouth, throat, and other cancers. Moreover, smoking impairs the ability of your immune system to perform one of its most important jobs—to destroy cancer cells.

Avoiding tobacco after a cancer diagnosis will

- improve your prognosis,

- lessen the likelihood of side effects from cancer treatments,

- reduce the likelihood of a recurrence of the cancer,

- and reduce your risk of developing a second cancer.

Clear evidence links tobacco use with cancers of the lung, mouth, throat, larynx, nasal passages, sinuses, esophagus, stomach, pancreas, kidney, bladder, uterine cervix, skin, and blood. Except for the relatively rare nasal and sinus cancers, these cancers are discussed below. Moreover, there is evidence that smoking may be implicated in the development of other cancers, particularly some colon, breast, anus, penis, vulvar, and liver cancers. Continuing research will likely reveal still other cancers linked to tobacco use.

Lung Cancer

23 Smoking causes 90 percent of lung cancer, a major killer.

Lung cancer kills far more Americans, both men and women, than any other type of cancer—about 160,000 a year. Smoking causes 90 percent of lung cancer cases. Women who smoke have a greater risk of lung cancer than men who have smoked an equal amount.

Lung cancer occurs mainly in smokers between the ages of 45 and 70. Consider the following:

- The younger you are when you begin smoking, the greater your risk of getting lung cancer.

- Your risk increases with the number of cigarettes you smoke each day, the number of years you smoke, and the amount of smoke you inhale.

- Someone who smokes two or more packs of cigarettes a day for 20 years has a 60 to 70 times greater risk of getting lung cancer than a person who has never smoked.

- When you quit smoking, your risk of getting lung cancer gradually decreases, even if you have smoked for decades.

- If you have been diagnosed with lung cancer you may live longer if you quit smoking.

As with other cancers, lung cancer occurs when cells begin to divide uncontrollably, forming masses of abnormal tissue and killing normal cells. Cough (especially coughing up reddish phlegm), shortness of breath, chest pain, fatigue, and weight loss are lung cancer symptoms that should be taken seriously. As lung cancer progresses, cancer cells often travel through the blood or the lymphatic system to start growths in other parts of the body, a process called *metastasis*.

The treatments for lung cancer include surgery, radiation therapy, and chemotherapy. Candidates for surgery have a much better five-year survival rate (about 50 percent) than those who cannot be treated surgically. Unfortunately, most lung cancers are not discovered early enough to be treated surgically. And surgery for lung cancer is a major operation. Surgery involves removing the tumor, part or all of the affected lung, and usually the lymph nodes into which the lung drains. Radiation therapy is sometimes used along with surgery. Several weeks or months may be needed for recuperation.

Emphysema, another deadly disease caused by smoking, sometimes afflicts those with lung cancer. Emphysema impedes the ability of the lungs to provide the body with oxygen. When a person with lung cancer also has emphysema, he or she may be unable to get enough oxygen if the cancerous lung is removed. For such patients surgery is not an option.

Patients with inoperable lung cancer can be treated with radiation therapy, chemotherapy, or a combination of the two. Radiation therapy consists of passing high-energy rays through the cancerous tissue. Chemotherapy consists of giving the patient anticancer drugs. The purpose of both is to destroy cancer cells or stop them from multiplying. Radiation therapy and chemotherapy may prolong the patient's life, but can have unpleasant side effects including nausea, vomiting, fatigue, temporary hair loss, and infection.

The overall survival rate for people diagnosed with lung cancer is dismally low. Only about 15 percent survive for five years. Although new treatments are being studied, the best way to avoid the pain, the unpleasantness, and the usually fatal outcome of lung cancer is to quit smoking or, better yet, not to start. With lung cancer, prevention is much more effective than treatment.

Cancers of the Mouth, Throat, and Larynx

24 **Tobacco use increases your chances of developing mouth or throat cancer. Nearly all mouth and throat cancers are found in people who use tobacco or abuse alcohol.**

In the United States, 90 percent of mouth and throat cancers are found in people who use some form of tobacco. People who abuse alcohol are also at risk. The combination of tobacco use and heavy drinking is especially likely to result in mouth or throat cancer. People who neither use tobacco nor drink alcohol—practicing Mormons, for example— almost never get mouth or throat cancer.

Mouth cancers can develop on the lip, tongue, gum, floor of the mouth, roof of the mouth, inside of the cheek, or salivary glands. If discovered and treated early, mouth cancer often can be cured, but more than half of mouth cancers are not discovered until they are advanced. Because of this, the five-year survival rate for people with mouth cancer is only about 50 percent.

Throat cancer occurs on the part of the throat just behind the mouth. The outlook for people with throat cancer varies considerably according to the site and the type of cancer, the stage of the disease when it is discovered, and the age of the person.

Surgery, radiation therapy, chemotherapy, or a combination, are used to treat mouth and throat cancer. Surgery may involve removal of all or parts of the jaw, tongue, teeth, or other structures, resulting in disfigurement that requires extensive plastic surgery. Problems with swallowing—and therefore with obtaining adequate nutrition—are also common, as are problems with speaking. Radiation therapy sometimes damages the salivary glands, resulting in a permanently dry mouth and difficulty swallowing, tasting, and speaking, as well as tooth decay.

About 8,000 Americans die of mouth or throat cancer each year. The surest way for you to avoid mouth or throat cancer is to avoid drinking excessive amounts of alcohol and to completely avoid tobacco. When you quit using tobacco, your risk of mouth or throat cancer drops substantially within three to five years. On the other hand, a person who contracts mouth or throat cancer has a nearly 40 percent risk of developing a second cancer if he or she does not quit using tobacco.

Cigarette, pipe, and cigar smokers are all at risk of mouth and throat cancer. Moreover, smokeless tobacco, such as chewing tobacco and moist snuff (finely ground tobacco that is held between the gum and cheek), is a major cause of mouth and throat cancer. The cancer usually occurs at the site where the tobacco is held. Unfortunately, as bans on public smoking increase and smokers are finding fewer places to smoke, some are turning to smokeless tobacco, rather than giving up tobacco altogether. Thus, the sales of smokeless tobacco have increased in recent years. Yet, as dangerous as smokeless tobacco is, it is less dangerous overall than smoking, and does not endanger other people by producing secondhand smoke.

25 If you smoke you run ten times the risk of cancer of the larynx as people who have never smoked.

Your *larynx,* or voice box, is located in the front of your neck just above the windpipe (the *trachea*). It contains vocal cords that produce the sounds of speech. Your larynx is also important to swallowing and breathing.

When you smoke cigarettes, cigars, or pipes, your larynx is directly exposed to the cancer-causing substances in tobacco. Smokers have about ten times the risk of cancer of the larynx as a person who has never smoked. If you drink excessive amounts of alcohol and smoke heavily, your larynx is at even greater risk of becoming cancerous. But the good news is that, if you stop drinking excessively and stop smoking, any precancerous cells in your larynx are likely to disappear.

Progressive hoarseness, breathlessness, persistent sore throat, and cough are symptoms of cancer of the larynx. Cancer of the larynx that is detected early can be cured without surgical removal of the larynx. But if the disease is advanced, removal of the larynx is often necessary. A patient without a larynx cannot speak normally, although technologies for voice synthesizing can help these patients communicate. A surgical procedure that leaves an open hole in the throat allows those without a larynx to push air through the esophagus and produce speech of sorts. Removal of the larynx also affects the ability to swallow. If the patient cannot swallow, a feeding tube may need to be implanted in the stomach through the abdominal wall.

If cancer of the larynx is far advanced, not even surgery can help. About 3,600 Americans die from cancer of the larynx each year. When you stop smoking, your risk of contracting cancer of the larynx begins to decline after three to four years. After ten years of abstinence from smoking, your risk approaches that of a person who has never smoked.

Other Cancers

26 **More than 40 percent of cancers of the esophagus and stomach are due to smoking, and the outlook for people with these cancers is usually poor.**

Preventing cancers of the esophagus and stomach is a far more effective strategy than treating them. Prevention includes a good diet, limited alcohol intake, and not using tobacco. According to new research, more than 40 percent of cancers of the esophagus and stomach are due to tobacco use.

Cancer of the esophagus is one of the most deadly of all cancers. It is also the fastest rising cancer in the United States. About 14,000 people die of cancer of the esophagus each year. Surgery can provide a cure in the early stages, but by the time there are symptoms the disease is usually advanced. Less than 13 percent of patients with advanced cancer of the esophagus survive five years.

Tobacco use of any type, including the use of smokeless tobacco, is a primary risk factor for cancer of the esophagus. Tobacco use is one cause of heartburn, the backing up of acidic stomach contents into the esophagus. If heartburn is frequent and severe, it can cause erosion and ulceration of the esophagus, leading to cancer.

The stomach is a sack-like organ just below the esophagus. Like cancer of the esophagus, stomach cancer usually produces no clear symptoms in its early stages, often spreading to distant sites before it is detected. Surgery offers the only chance for a cure of stomach cancer and, when surgery is indicated, part or all of the stomach may have to be removed, severely restricting food intake. However, in 80 percent of cases the stomach cancer is too far advanced for surgical treatment. Only ten percent of patients with inoperable stomach cancer survive longer than five years. In the United States, about 11,000 people die of stomach cancer each year. Not smoking will significantly decrease your risk of this disease.

27 Smoking is an important cause of pancreatic cancer, a deadly disease with few survivors.

Your pancreas is a large gland that lies behind your stomach. Your pancreas secretes insulin and glucagon, hormones that work together to maintain proper blood glucose (sugar) levels. Your pancreas also secretes enzymes that digest food in the small intestine.

Cancer of the pancreas is the fourth most deadly cancer, killing about 34,000 Americans each year. Early diagnosis is difficult because the disease typically produces no symptoms until it has spread, making a cure impossible. Only two percent of patients are still alive five years after diagnosis.

Cancer of the pancreas is two to three times more common in people who smoke heavily than in nonsmokers. Other risk factors are chronic pancreatitis (a long-standing inflammation of the pancreas, often caused by alcoholism), certain inherited gene mutations, obesity, physical inactivity, and periodontal (gum) disease. Former smokers are at somewhat lower risk of cancer of the pancreas than smokers, although it may take ten or more smoke-free years to reduce the risk substantially. The sooner you stop smoking, the lower your risk of contracting cancer of the pancreas.

28 Smoking increases your risk of developing kidney cancer by 40 percent.

Your kidneys are a pair of bean-shaped organs weighing about six ounces each. They lie in the back of your abdomen, just above the waist. The functions of your kidneys are essential to life. Your kidneys filter your blood, removing waste materials and excess water, and return nutrients into your blood. The waste materials and excess water (urine) flow from each kidney down its ureter, a tube that delivers urine to the urinary bladder.

More than 50,000 cases of kidney cancer are diagnosed each year in this country and more than 12,000 people die from it. The symptoms of kidney cancer include blood in the urine, pain in the side, intermittent fever, weight loss, and fatigue. Kidney cancer usually occurs in people over age 40, and is twice as common in men as in women.

In some instances, kidney cancer appears to be inherited. Studies show that a diet low in fruits and vegetables and high in fats may be a risk factor. However, smoking is the most important risk factor for kidney cancer. Smoking increases your risk of developing kidney cancer by 40 percent. And the longer you smoke, the higher your risk. If you quit smoking, you'll begin to reduce your risk of kidney cancer within just a few years.

29 **Cigarette smoking is by far the most important cause of bladder cancer, accounting for 25 percent of cases in women and 50 percent in men.**

Your urinary bladder is a hollow organ that receives urine from your kidneys and stores it until it is discharged through the urethra. In the United States, an estimated 57,000 new cases of bladder cancer are diagnosed each year. Bladder cancer is often detected during a routine urinalysis screening, before symptoms appear. But in other cases, people seek treatment because of bloody urine, or pain or burning when urinating.

About 75 percent of bladder cancers are superficial tumors growing on the inside wall of the bladder, but not deep into the wall. These cancers can be removed surgically, and 90 percent of patients survive, but recurrence of the cancer is common.

Those cancers that have grown deep into the bladder wall are usually treated by radiation therapy and by removing the entire bladder or a portion of it—along with the prostate in men, and the ovaries, womb, and part of the vagina in women. An artificial bladder can be made from a piece of intestine.

Bladder cancer that has spread to other organs requires chemotherapy, but only a small percentage of these patients can be cured. In the United States, bladder cancer causes nearly 14,000 deaths each year.

Cigarette smoking is by far the most important cause of bladder cancer. Cancer-causing chemicals in cigarette smoke enter the bloodstream, are filtered out by the kidneys, and pass into urine that is stored in the bladder. The more cigarettes per day that you smoke and the more years you have smoked, the greater your risk of bladder cancer. But if you quit smoking your risk will gradually decrease.

30 Women infected with certain strains of human papilloma virus greatly increase their risk of cervical cancer by smoking.

The uterus, or womb, is a pear-shaped organ with the narrow end, the cervix, at the bottom. The cervix opens into the vagina, permitting the passage of menstrual fluid from the uterus, and the passage of sperm into the uterus. During childbirth, the cervix opens wide so that the baby can pass through the vagina.

Cervical cancer occurs most often in women between the ages of 30 and 55 years. It was a leading cause of death in American women before the development in the 1940s of a test, called the Pap smear, that can detect it in its early stages. Because cervical cancer develops slowly, women who have Pap smears on a regular basis can nearly always be cured, often by relatively simple procedures.

Unfortunately, about 40 percent of American women do not have regular Pap smears, and there typically is no pain or other symptom in cervical cancer's early stages. Of women with advanced cervical cancer, about 4,000 a year die within five years of diagnosis. Even if an advanced cervical cancer is detected in time to save the woman's life, treatment can involve removal of the uterus, ovaries, and part of the vagina.

Women who develop cervical cancer usually are infected with certain strains of *human papilloma virus* (HPV). HPV is transmitted through sexual activity. Therefore, risk factors for cervical cancer include having multiple sex partners, or a sex partner who has had multiple sex partners. Fortunately, a vaccine that will prevent infection with human papilloma virus has recently been developed. But this vaccine must be given *before* infection occurs. The vaccine cannot treat an existing infection. It is therefore most effective if given before young people become sexually active. The Centers for Disease Control recommends that girls eleven and twelve be vaccinated.

Like HPV, smoking is a risk factor for cervical cancer. Cancer-promoting chemicals in cigarette smoke travel through the bloodstream and can be found in the cervical secretions of smokers. A recent study found that women smokers infected with HVP are 14 times more likely to develop cervical cancer than infected nonsmokers. But after two years of abstaining from smoking, a woman's risk of developing cervical cancer is the same as a nonsmoker's.

31 Smoking increases your risk of getting the type of skin cancer known as squamous cell carcinoma. It also increases your risk of dying if you get malignant melanoma, another type of skin cancer.

Skin cancer occurs more frequently than any other type of human cancer. Your chances of getting skin cancer are greater if you are fair-skinned or have had a great deal of sun exposure. Smoking adds to your risk of developing the type of skin cancer called *squamous cell carcinoma*, and to the likelihood of your dying if you get another type of skin cancer called *malignant melanoma*.

Squamous cell carcinoma is one of the most common types of skin cancer. It is a slow-growing cancer but, if left untreated, it can be fatal. Most of the medical studies that have evaluated smoking as a risk factor for getting squamous cell carcinoma have concluded that smokers are at greater risk than nonsmokers. Consider the following:

- One large study indicated a 50 percent greater risk for smokers.

- A recent study found that people who smoke 11 to 20 cigarettes a day have three times the risk of nonsmokers, and those who smoke more than 20 cigarettes have four times the risk.

- Another study found that smokers who have experienced an initial incidence of squamous cell carcinoma, and who continue to smoke, are twice as likely as lifelong nonsmokers to experience it a second time.

- While sun exposure is a contributing factor to squamous cell carcinoma of the lip, 80 percent of the people who develop this particular cancer are smokers.

Malignant melanoma is less common than squamous cell carcinoma, but more deadly. Malignant melanoma originates in the cells of the skin that produce melanin, the pigment that gives color to the skin. Environmental damage to the protective ozone layer of the earth's atmosphere may have contributed to the increase of this type of skin cancer in recent years. Malignant melanoma currently claims over

8,000 lives in the United States annually, despite a high cure rate with early detection.

Smoking does not cause malignant melanoma. But smokers who contract malignant melanoma are more likely to die of it. The body's immune system, working together with anti-melanoma vaccines and other drugs, is key to fighting advanced malignant melanoma. Smoking impairs the immune system, thus reducing its ability to fight this disease.

32 If you smoke, you run a greater risk of contracting acute myeloid leukemia, a cancer of the blood cells.

Leukemia is cancer of the blood cells. Abnormal white blood cells accumulate in the blood and bone marrow, causing fatigue, weakness, fever, pallor, a tendency to bleed or bruise easily, loss of appetite, and bone pain, among other symptoms. Leukemia occurs more often in men than in women, and is the fifth most deadly cancer for men.

Leukemia can progress slowly (*chronic leukemia*) or rapidly (*acute leukemia*). Untreated, acute leukemia kills in a few weeks or months. Cigarette smoking causes about one in five cases of one type of acute leukemia, *acute myeloid leukemia*. Some scientists believe that benzene, one of the chemicals in tobacco smoke, is responsible. Exposure to benzene is a known cause of acute myeloid leukemia. Studies indicate that heavy smokers have a greater risk of contracting this leukemia than those who smoke fewer cigarettes.

About 13,400 cases of acute myeloid leukemia are diagnosed yearly in the United States, mostly in adults.

Although some patients respond to treatment with chemotherapy or bone marrow transplantation, they are often extremely ill before they get better. The five-year survival rate is about 33 percent for patients under 65 and four percent for patients over 65. Smokers' increased risk of contracting acute myeloid leukemia provides another good reason not to smoke.

LUNG DISEASES

Emphysema, Chronic Bronchitis, and Asthma

33 **Smoking causes most cases of emphysema, a tormenting and often fatal lung disease with no cure.**

Emphysema is a progressively crippling lung disease that is usually caused by smoking. The *alveoli*—tiny air sacs in the lungs—deliver oxygen to the blood and remove carbon dioxide from it. Emphysema develops gradually as smoking causes more and more of these air sacs to rupture. As the emphysema progresses, the lungs become less elastic, which limits their ability to function properly.

The first symptoms of emphysema may not appear until your 50s or 60s. By then, 50 percent or more of your lung tissues may be damaged. Quitting when symptoms appear will slow emphysema's further progress. But the damage already done is irreversible. Not quitting almost guarantees that you'll spend the rest of your life struggling to breathe or tethered to an oxygen source, with an increasingly compromised quality of life. People with severe emphysema are often confined to wheelchair and bed. Depression is common in these people. Many die from heart failure.

In addition to increasing shortness of breath, emphysema sufferers may experience a persistent cough. They often fall victim to respiratory infections. When chronic bronchitis accompanies emphysema—which is usually the case—the combination is called *chronic obstructive pulmonary disease* (COPD). Doctors strongly urge people diagnosed with emphysema or COPD to stop smoking and to avoid other lung irritants, such as secondhand tobacco smoke, that can worsen the condition.

Avoiding tobacco smoke may greatly improve the stamina and symptoms of a person who has been diagnosed with emphysema. Pulmonary rehabilitation programs are education and exercise programs designed to help people with emphysema live with their disease. Some of these programs also help participants quit smoking. A person with emphysema who has participated in a rehabilitation program and has quit smoking may be a candidate for lung volume reduction surgery. This surgery can improve quality of life for emphysema patients.

34 If you smoke, you are 20 times more likely than a nonsmoker to develop chronic bronchitis, a progressively disabling disease that can lead to heart failure.

Your trachea, or windpipe, is a tube extending down through your neck into your chest cavity. There it branches into the right and left bronchi, which further divide and subdivide into smaller and smaller branches that penetrate deep within your lungs. The bronchi and their branches are called the bronchial tubes. They provide the passageway for air in and out of the lungs. Bronchitis is an inflammation of the bronchial tubes caused by infection or irritants. Inflammation of the bronchial tubes generates increased mucus, which clogs the airways and must be coughed up.

There are two types of bronchitis: acute and chronic. A respiratory infection, such as a cold, strep throat, or influenza, sometimes extends down into the bronchial tubes, causing *acute bronchitis*. The irritants in cigarette smoke also can cause acute bronchitis. Acute bronchitis is often characterized by a cough that brings up thick yellow or gray mucus. For healthy nonsmokers, acute bronchitis ordinarily is not dangerous, and with rest it usually goes away within a week or so. But smoking irritates the lining of the bronchial tubes and paralyzes the cilia, hairlike projections in the bronchial tubes that sweep the airways free of mucus and debris. Therefore, if you smoke you are at risk of repeated attacks of acute bronchitis and of developing *chronic bronchitis*.

Unlike acute bronchitis, chronic bronchitis does not go away. A person with chronic bronchitis typically has a long history of cigarette smoking—indeed, if you smoke you are 20 times more likely than a nonsmoker to develop chronic bronchitis. A smoker who is exposed to smog, or to fumes or smoke in the workplace, has an even greater risk of developing chronic bronchitis.

Chronic bronchitis is characterized by a persistent cough that brings up thick mucus, and by repeated respiratory infections. The bronchial tubes are inflamed and thickened, narrowing the passage for air. Shortness of breath and wheezing eventually become evident and are progressively disabling. A person with chronic bronchitis usually has emphysema also. When the two diseases occur together, the condition is called chronic obstructive pulmonary disease, or COPD. In the United States, COPD ranks fourth as a cause of death.

Advanced chronic bronchitis often leads to *cor pulmonale,* the enlargement and failure of the right chamber of the heart due to poor lung function. People with cor pulmonale may have bluish skin, lips, and nails due to a lack of oxygen. They may retain fluid and have swollen feet, legs, and hands. Chronic bronchitis by itself can kill, but death from heart failure is a more usual outcome.

If you are a smoker who has developed chronic bronchitis, and you quit smoking, the progress of the disease can be halted. But clearly, the better choice is to prevent chronic bronchitis by quitting before it develops.

35 Smoking worsens the chronic bronchial inflammation of asthma and triggers acute asthma attacks.

Worldwide, the incidence of asthma has been on the rise. In the United States, seven percent of people have asthma and about 5,000 die of it each year. Although asthma is sometimes thought of as a children's disease, it can develop at any age. Eleven million American adults have asthma.

Asthma is a lung disease marked by chronic inflammation of the bronchial tubes (the air passages in the lungs) and unpredictable acute attacks of breathlessness, wheezing, coughing, and tightness in the chest that may last for a few minutes—or for several days if the attack is especially severe. An acute asthma attack is caused by narrowing of the bronchial tubes. This happens when the bronchial tubes constrict, become clogged with mucus, or when the membranes lining them become swollen. Although acute asthma attacks are more often uncomfortable and frightening than dangerous, during a severe attack the bronchial tubes may collapse, causing suffocation if the person does not receive immediate medical care.

Someone with asthma has bronchial tubes that are hypersensitive to certain allergens (often house dust, pollens, animal dander, feathers, wool, or mold) or to irritants, such as fumes or smoke. Tobacco smoke worsens the chronic bronchial inflammation of asthma. It is also one of the most common triggers of acute asthma attacks because it irritates the bronchial tubes, making them prone to constrict. Tobacco smoke exposure makes babies more likely to get asthma.

Although chronic inflammation and acute constriction of the bronchial tubes can be controlled with medication, exposure to tobacco smoke reduces the effectiveness of asthma medications. Moreover, a smoker may develop chronic bronchitis or emphysema. These diseases complicate asthma. If you have asthma, it is vital that you not smoke and not allow smoking in your home.

Influenza, Pneumonia, and Tuberculosis

36 **Smoking puts you at greater risk of contracting influenza and pneumonia and makes you more likely to die from these diseases.**

Influenza (flu) is a highly contagious infection of the air passages caused by a virus. A person with flu usually has a fever, headache, muscle aches, and fatigue—and often a cough, sore throat, and runny nose. The serious threat is not flu itself, as unpleasant as that can be, but rather the profound weakness flu causes that can result in a bacterial infection, especially pneumonia. Flu also can worsen chronic diseases such as diabetes, and heart, lung, and kidney ailments. Every year about 36,000 Americans die from complications of flu.

Because smoking paralyzes the cilia, hairlike cells that help clear the nasal and lung passages of viruses and bacteria, smokers have a greater risk of contracting flu. The suppression of the immune system that smoking causes may also be a factor. There is an annual vaccine against flu that is 70 to 90 percent effective, but smokers derive less immunity from it than nonsmokers. And a smoker's flu is more likely than a nonsmoker's to progress to pneumonia.

Pneumonia is a possible complication of flu or any other serious illness. Someone with pneumonia has inflamed lungs, usually due to infection by bacteria or viruses. Parts of the lungs fill with fluid that clogs the lungs' tiny air sacs (alveoli) and prevents oxygen from reaching the blood. Typical symptoms of pneumonia are chest pain, chills and fever, and shortness of breath, along with a cough that brings up yellow-green mucus and sometimes blood. Pneumonia ranges in severity from mild to life threatening. It is the sixth leading cause of death in this country.

Young, healthy people usually overcome pneumonia and, indeed, often regard it as merely a bad cold. Pneumonia is much more dangerous for people with heart failure, chronic bronchitis, emphysema, cancer, or asthma. Smoking often causes these diseases or makes them worse, which is one reason that smokers have a higher death rate from pneumonia than nonsmokers. But even a smoker who has none of these diseases runs a greater risk of contracting pneumonia, for the same reasons that he's more susceptible to influenza. One study finds smokers three times more likely to contract pneumonia than nonsmokers. Moreover, a smoker's pneumonia is more likely to be severe or fatal than a nonsmoker's. In 2008, the federal Advisory Committee on Immunization Practices recommended that adult smokers under 65 years old get a vaccination that protects against pneumonia. Previously, only people over 65 were advised to get this vaccination.

When you quit smoking, your susceptibility to influenza and pneumonia gradually decreases. People who smoke heavily must abstain for about 15 years before their risk of death from influenza and pneumonia approaches that of nonsmokers; light smokers must abstain for about ten years.

37 If you smoke and have dormant tuberculosis, you are two and one-half times more likely than a nonsmoker to get active tuberculosis.

Tuberculosis is a disease caused by infection with tuberculosis bacteria. It kills more people worldwide than any other infectious disease—more than three million each year. An important symptom of active tuberculosis is a cough. Tuberculosis is spread when a person with active tuberculosis coughs, expelling droplets containing tuberculosis bacteria into air that other people inhale. In most infected people the tuberculosis bacteria lie dormant in the body and never develop into an active disease. But tuberculosis can become active if the immune system is weakened. Treatment of active tuberculosis involves antibiotics taken over many months. Unfortunately, a few people develop drug-resistant strains of tuberculosis that cannot be cured with antibiotics.

Although tuberculosis can affect other organs in the body, it usually affects the lungs. Smoking weakens the lungs' defenses and is a risk factor for activating tuberculosis. If you smoke and have dormant tuberculosis, you are two and one-half times more likely than a nonsmoker to get active tuberculosis. And when smokers get active tuberculosis, it generally is more severe than it is in nonsmokers. Moreover, a smoker may confuse a cough caused by tuberculosis with a cigarette cough, resulting in delayed treatment—while the smoker spreads tuberculosis to family members, friends, coworkers, and other people that the smoker has contact with.

Other Lung Problems

38 **A smoker is much more likely than a nonsmoker to suffer a collapsed lung.**

A *collapsed lung* occurs when air gets into the *pleural space*—the space between the lung and the chest wall—compressing or collapsing the lung. Air in the pleural space ranges in seriousness from a condition so minor that you may not even notice it, to a life-threatening emergency. Chest injury—sustained in an automobile crash, for example—sometimes causes a lung to collapse. Or a weak point may develop in the lung of a young person, usually a male smoker between the ages of 20 and 40. If the weak point ruptures, allowing air to enter the pleural space, the lung collapses.

Older smokers, especially those who have lung diseases caused or made worse by smoking (chronic bronchitis, emphysema, or asthma), are much more likely than nonsmokers to suffer a collapsed lung. Smoking weakens the lungs, making them more susceptible to rupture. Once you have had a collapsed lung, you run a 50 percent risk of getting another, in which case surgery is often necessary. Doctors strongly advise anyone who has had a collapsed lung to stop smoking.

39 Everyone's lung function declines with age, but in smokers this decline is more rapid than in nonsmokers.

With good lung function, you have elastic lungs with lung capacity (the amount of air the lungs can hold) normal for your age, sex, and height. Good lung function also requires that there be no narrowing or blockage of the airways. How well your lungs function can be determined by a test using a machine called a spirometer. First, you inhale as deeply as possible, then exhale as hard and fast as possible into the spirometer.

Everyone's lung function declines with age, but in smokers this decline is more rapid than in nonsmokers. However, when you quit smoking you regain lung function, and your decline in lung function slows down. Eventually, you will have an annual decline in lung function similar to that of a person who has never smoked.

40 Chronic shortness of breath is much more likely if you smoke—and there is no guarantee that it will disappear when you quit.

Shortness of breath, or breathlessness, is normal in someone who is exercising vigorously or otherwise exerting himself. However, if you develop shortness of breath for any other reason, it is an indication of an underlying disorder and calls for a visit to your doctor. Smokers have a greater incidence of chronic shortness of breath than people who have never smoked.

Heart disease, which is more common in smokers, can cause chronic shortness of breath. Moreover, smoking begins damaging the lungs with the first cigarette. A smoker with chronic shortness of breath may already have significant lung damage. Unfortunately, a smoker's chronic shortness of breath often does not disappear when he or she stops smoking. Chronic shortness of breath can greatly compromise your quality of life. The risk of developing chronic shortness of breath is a good reason not to start smoking, or to stop smoking before it develops.

41 Many smokers develop a constant, annoying cigarette cough that can interfere with sleep, work, and social life.

Coughing, a necessary and protective reflex, is your body's attempt to rid your lungs or throat of foreign material. A cough also can be a symptom of an illness, such as a cold, flu, laryngitis, bronchitis, emphysema, pneumonia, tuberculosis, or lung cancer.

Many smokers develop a constant, annoying "cigarette cough." Tobacco smoke irritates the throat and bronchial tubes, sometimes causing a dry cough—that is, a cough that does not produce sputum. Sputum is matter ejected from the respiratory tract, matter that contains mucus (phlegm), pus, cellular debris, microorganisms, foreign materials, or blood. Smokers also may have a productive cough—a cough that does produce sputum—especially on arising in the morning. Abnormally large amounts of thick sputum in breathing passages inflamed by tobacco smoke trigger a smoker's productive cough. A chronic smoker's cough that changes in frequency or character is a warning that medical attention is needed.

A cigarette cough can interfere with your work and social life. You may feel exhausted because coughing takes a lot of energy and interferes with your sleep. A harsh or forceful cough can further irritate your breathing passages, helping to perpetuate the cough. Violent coughing can cause a sore throat, urinary incontinence, or even vomiting, rib fractures, a hernia (a protrusion of part of the intestine through the abdominal wall), or uterine prolapse (descent of the womb into the vagina).

Ironically, a cigarette cough may get worse for a short time after you quit smoking. The function of the cilia, tiny hairs lining the breathing passages, is to propel sputum up to be expelled, but tobacco smoke paralyzes the cilia. A person who has recently quit smoking may have a hacking cough as the cilia—no longer paralyzed—work hard to get rid of trapped debris. Over time, though, the coughing should lessen. Studies indicate that cough and sputum production usually decline when people quit smoking, regardless of the length of time they smoked or the amount they smoked.

42 Smokers get more colds and longer-lasting colds than nonsmokers, display more severe cold symptoms, and develop secondary bacterial infections more readily.

The common cold is a viral infection that can be caused by any of 200 different viruses spread through the air, or by contact with surfaces touched by someone who already has a cold. If you smoke, you are more likely to catch frequent colds. Your colds are likely to be more severe and last longer than if you didn't smoke. And you are more apt to develop a serious secondary bacterial infection, such as sinusitis, middle-ear infection, laryngitis, bronchitis, or even pneumonia.

Smokers are more susceptible to colds because tobacco smoke paralyzes the cilia, hairlike cells in the nasal and lung passages that normally sweep out infectious viruses and bacteria. Tobacco smoke also may reduce the effectiveness of the protective mucus barrier that lines your respiratory tract. And smoking impairs your immune system, lowering your resistance to viral and secondary bacterial infections.

Colds generally make you feel miserable enough to want to stay home in bed. And if you smoke during a cold, the added irritation to your already inflamed nasal and throat passages will make you feel worse.

43 If you have hay fever you should avoid inhaling irritants, such as tobacco smoke, that will make the hay fever worse.

Ordinarily, your immune system protects you from harmful bacteria, viruses, and other infectious agents. An allergy is an overreaction of your immune system to a normally harmless substance. Substances that cause allergies are called *allergens. Allergic rhinitis,* commonly called hay fever, is an allergic reaction triggered by inhaled allergens. The allergens that cause most cases of hay fever are pollens, molds, house dust, and animal dander. Hay fever afflicts up to 40 million Americans each year.

While hay fever rarely causes disability, it can be an extreme nuisance, causing nasal congestion with a watery discharge, watering of the eyes, itching and irritation of the nose and eyes, throat irritation, and sneezing. Some families seem to be more susceptible to allergies than others, so hay fever is believed to be partly hereditary.

Avoiding the offending allergen (or allergens) as much as possible provides some relief, and medications can help control uncomfortable symptoms. Allergy shots make some sufferers less sensitive to the inhaled substance that is causing the allergic reaction.

If you have hay fever you should also avoid inhaled irritants that make the condition worse. These include industrial smoke, face powder, powdered laundry detergents, and tobacco smoke. In a few people, tobacco smoke itself is the allergen causing the hay fever. Avoiding tobacco smoke is essential in these cases.

BRAIN AND NERVE DISEASES

Dementias and Schizophrenia

44 Smoking is a risk factor for Alzheimer's disease and vascular dementia.

Dementia is a chronic, slowly progressive illness resulting in loss of mental functioning. *Alzheimer's disease* is the most common type of dementia. *Vascular dementia* is the second most common, afflicting 20 percent of people with dementia.

The incidence of Alzheimer's disease rises sharply with advancing age, reaching almost 50 percent in people over 85. It always ends in death and is the seventh leading cause of death in the elderly. There is no cure, although medications may slow the progression of the disease.

Fortunately, there are steps that can be taken to help prevent Alzheimer's disease. These include engaging in regular physical and mental exercise, keeping blood pressure under control, raising good cholesterol and lowering bad cholesterol, maintaining a healthy weight, eating a healthy diet, preventing or controlling diabetes, keeping alcohol consumption moderate, taking statin medications, and not smoking. One study showed that current smokers were almost three times as likely to develop Alzheimer's disease as nonsmokers. So if you worry about developing Alzheimer's disease, then don't smoke.

Smoking is a major risk factor for the second most common dementia—vascular dementia. Vascular dementia usually results from loss of blood supply to the brain due to narrowed or blocked arteries. In some cases, the dementia begins after a major stroke. But in many cases, multiple small strokes gradually destroy brain tissue. Therefore, vascular dementia is also called *multi-infarct dementia*. (An infarct is tissue that dies when its blood supply is cut off.) This series of small strokes may leave little or no immediate weakness or paralysis, as is often the case with a major stroke. Unlike Alzheimer's disease, in vascular dementia mental deterioration usually happens in a step-wise pattern.

High blood pressure and atherosclerosis (plaque deposits in arteries) are major causes of vascular dementia. Smoking makes high blood pressure worse and is a risk factor for atherosclerosis. Smoking also increases the risk of blood clots. The most common cause of stroke is a blood clot that blocks a blood vessel supplying the brain with blood.

Not smoking and careful control of high blood pressure help prevent vascular dementia. Patients diagnosed with vascular dementia can reduce their risk of additional strokes if they quit smoking.

45 Smokers have much higher rates of schizophrenia than nonsmokers.

Schizophrenia is a psychotic disorder with symptoms that may include delusions, hallucinations, disorganized speech, catatonia (muscular rigidity or excessive physical agitation), or withdrawal from social interaction. A schizophrenic person may have an inability to feel pleasure or happiness, or have a blunting of normal emotional responses.

People with schizophrenia smoke cigarettes at startlingly high rates. Up to 90 percent of schizophrenics are smokers, and they are among the heaviest smokers. Some experts believe schizophrenics self-medicate with cigarettes, while others believe that smoking may cause schizophrenia. One study showed that adolescents who smoked were more likely to develop schizophrenia than adolescents who did not smoke.

People with schizophrenia are less able to cope with smoking-related diseases than are mentally healthy people. But, fortunately, the mentally ill are able to quit smoking, especially if they have help from their doctors.

Depression and Suicide

46 Depression and suicide is more common among smokers than among nonsmokers.

Depression is a serious illness that makes life miserable. Occasional feelings of sadness are normal, but depression is not normal sadness. A depressed person usually loses interest in the pleasures of life such as food, sex, entertainment, sports, work, and hobbies. Recent studies indicate that chronic depression may actually cause a heart attack or hasten death. People who are depressed cannot get over it by willpower alone. Fortunately, doctors can prescribe safe and effective drugs to treat depression.

The relationship between smoking and depression is uncertain and complex. Some experts believe that smoking causes depression by affecting brain chemicals. Others believe that depressed people begin smoking and continue to smoke because they are "self-medicating" their depression with cigarettes. The experts do agree that smokers have a much higher rate of depression than nonsmokers.

If smoking causes depression, that is certainly another compelling reason not to smoke. If, on the other hand, smokers self-medicate their depression with cigarettes, it is hard to imagine a worse choice of medication. Cigarettes can have terrible side effects, including lung cancer, heart disease, emphysema, and the many other illnesses discussed in this book. Treating depression with one of the antidepressant medications now available is a much wiser choice. Moreover, antidepressants can help you stop smoking whether or not you are depressed.

In extreme cases, depression leads to suicide. Suicide claims the lives of about 30,000 Americans each year. It is a tragedy that usually impacts not only the suicide victim, but many other people as well. Those close to the victim may feel a grief greater than they would have if the death had been from natural causes. They may feel guilt, remorse, and shame because they were unable to prevent the suicide. Family members of a suicide victim are at greater risk of suicide themselves.

Smoking has been called "slow suicide," but smokers are at increased risk of "quick suicide," as well. Numerous studies of people who have committed suicide show that smokers are much more likely to kill themselves than nonsmokers. For example:

- A study of more than 100,000 American nurses found that, compared to those who had never smoked, those who smoked one to 24 cigarettes a day had twice the risk of suicide, and those who smoked 25 or more cigarettes had four times the risk.

■ A study of 300,000 male soldiers on active duty in the U.S. Army found that soldiers who smoked more than 20 cigarettes a day were more than twice as likely to commit suicide, compared to those soldiers who had never smoked. These researchers also found that the more the soldiers smoked, the greater their risk of suicide.

■ More than 50,000 middle-aged and elderly male health professionals were followed in another study. These researchers found that, compared to those who had never smoked, the risk of suicide was 40 percent higher for former smokers, 250 percent higher for light smokers, and 450 percent higher for heavy smokers.

There are many reasons why smokers are more likely to commit suicide. Depression is a factor in the majority of suicides and we know that depression is much more common in smokers than in nonsmokers. Physical illnesses—especially those illnesses that are serious, chronic, or painful—play a role in many suicides. Smokers are at greater risk of developing devastating illnesses such as heart disease, cancer, and emphysema. Alcohol abuse is also a factor in many suicides. Smokers are more likely than nonsmokers to abuse alcohol. Unmarried people have a greater tendency than married people to commit suicide, and smokers are more likely than nonsmokers to be single. Fortunately, former smokers have a lower risk of suicide than current smokers, another good reason to quit smoking.

Stress and Anxiety

47 Smoking increases your stress, even though you may believe that you smoke to relieve stress.

We experience stress when our ability to adapt is over-whelmed by events. Circumstances that cause stress are called *stressors*. The death of a spouse, a divorce, a personal injury or illness, being fired from a job, or an adverse change in finances are major stressors. Stressors may persist over a long period of time—for example, an unhappy marriage, a hated job, or involvement in wartime combat. The accelerating change of modern life increases stress. Even joyous events, such as getting married, the birth of a child, or a job promotion, cause stress. Smaller, everyday events add stress, too—rushing to make an appointment, your child's cold, or sitting in traffic.

People differ greatly in their reactions to stressors but, generally speaking, the more stressors you are subjected to, the more serious the stressors, and the longer you are subjected to them, the more likely they are to damage your health. Chronic severe stress can damage the immune system and contribute to the development of heart disease, high blood pressure, diabetes, headaches, anxiety disorders, indigestion, skin rashes, impotence, and other health problems. Chronic stress also increases the likelihood of accidents. Smoking, and the guilt and worry that often accompany smoking, increase chronic stress.

The relationship between stress and smoking is complex. Some experts believe that many young people begin smoking in an attempt to relieve the stress associated with adolescence. And smokers usually believe that smoking relieves stress. However, studies have found that the only stress smoking relieves is the stress caused by nicotine addiction itself. A smoker who has not had a cigarette for a while begins to experience stress from nicotine withdrawal. Smoking relieves that stress, but stress begins to build again as soon as the cigarette is stubbed out. Thus, a smoker goes through daylong cycles of stress from nicotine withdrawal, followed by temporary relief when he or she has a cigarette.

Studies have determined that both nonsmokers and former smokers feel less stress than smokers. However, quitting smoking is often quite stressful. Some smokers are able to tolerate the stress of quitting suddenly, but most benefit from gradual withdrawal using nicotine patches, lozenges, or chewing gum. The support provided by a smoking cessation clinic helps many smokers through the stressful period of quitting. While you are trying to quit, just remember that the period of increased stress is *temporary,* and you will have less stress for the rest of your life if you are successful.

48 Smoking makes anxiety disorders worse.

It is normal to feel anxiety about real problems, but someone who has irrational or excessive anxiety is said to have an anxiety disorder. There are several types of anxiety disorders. *Generalized anxiety disorder* is the most common. People with this condition feel anxious most of the time, usually without any real cause. A second type of anxiety disorder is *phobia,* an uncontrollable, irrational, persistent fear of something—for example, a fear of dogs, elevators, flying, thunder, public speaking, or crowds.

A third type of anxiety is *panic disorder,* which causes sudden feelings of terror for no apparent reason. Breathlessness, dizziness, trembling, sweating, nausea, heart palpitations, or feelings of unreality may accompany a panic attack. Panic attacks often lead to a phobia called *agoraphobia*, a fear of situations or places in which the panic attacks have occurred.

Yet another type of anxiety disorder is *obsessive-compulsive disorder*. An obsession is a seemingly senseless idea, image, impulse, or thought that keeps recurring. A compulsion is an act that a person with an obsession performs to dispel the anxiety that the obsession causes. For example, a man who is obsessed with germs may feel a compulsion to continually wash his hands. A woman who is obsessed with the thought that she has hit someone with her automobile may feel a compulsion to continually check the rear view mirror to make sure that this has not happened.

Post-traumatic stress disorder is another anxiety disorder. It was first identified in soldiers during World War I, when it was called "shell shock." But post-traumatic stress disorder can occur in any person who has experienced an event that caused terror or feelings of helplessness. Such events include airplane or automobile crashes, rape, assault, torture, tornadoes, and earthquakes—as well as wartime combat. A person with post-traumatic stress disorder may suffer repetitive, distressing thoughts about the experience, feelings that the experience is recurring, and nightmares. These and other reactions may occur for months or years.

Anxiety disorders are treated with medications and various types of therapy. Physicians and psychologists advise people with anxiety disorders to avoid caffeine and nicotine—both are stimulants that worsen anxiety. Although smokers usually believe that smoking calms their nerves, studies show that the opposite is true. Smokers tend to be more anxious than nonsmokers.

One study found that teenagers who smoke a pack or more a day run a greatly increased risk of developing anxiety disorders as young adults. Compared to teenagers who do not smoke, their risk of generalized anxiety disorder is 5.5 times greater, of agoraphobia 6.8 times greater, and of panic disorder 15.5 times greater. People who quit smoking become less prone to anxiety and panic.

Of course, smokers have a well-founded cause for anxiety that nonsmokers don't have. Many are anxious about the harm that smoking is doing to their health and the harm their secondhand smoke is doing to others. Fortunately, this anxiety helps many smokers commit themselves to quitting.

49 Hyperventilation is usually caused by anxiety, and smoking increases anxiety.

Hyperventilation is overbreathing—that is, breathing too much. When you hyperventilate, you lose too much carbon dioxide from your blood. Paradoxically, you then feel as if you are suffocating and may breathe harder, making the problem worse. During hyperventilation, faintness and tingling sensations in the fingers, toes, or lips are sometimes accompanied by a feeling of impending doom. The usual treatment for hyperventilation is shutting the mouth and pinching off one nostril so that less oxygen is taken in and the level of carbon dioxide in the blood is normalized. Although hyperventilation is not dangerous, it can be extremely distressing. It may also be a symptom of an underlying disease, such as asthma, emphysema, congestive heart failure, or heart attack. Therefore, a person who has never before experienced hyperventilation should seek medical attention.

However, the most common cause of hyperventilation is anxiety. Stimulants, such as nicotine in tobacco, can increase anxiety. If you are a smoker who is subject to attacks of hyperventilation due to anxiety, quitting smoking will make you less likely to have such attacks.

Lou Gehrig's Disease

50 Smokers are at increased risk of contracting Lou Gehrig's disease (ALS), a devastating and fatal illness.

Amyotrophic lateral sclerosis (ALS) is popularly known as "Lou Gehrig's disease" after the famous baseball player who contracted this devastating illness. ALS attacks nerve cells in the brain and spinal cord. The disease causes progressive loss of muscle control. Muscles waste away and, in the later stages of ALS, the person becomes completely paralyzed, unable to swallow, or to breathe without a respirator. Patients usually survive three to five years, although a few live ten years or even longer.

About 30,000 Americans have ALS at any given time. Five to ten percent of cases are inherited. The cause of the other cases is unknown. There is no cure for ALS, but new treatment appears to prolong life by several months.

Recent research has concluded that smoking increases your risk of contracting ALS. The findings in one study indicate that *ever* having smoked almost doubles your risk. Another study indicates a greater than threefold increased risk for current smokers.

DIGESTIVE TRACT DISEASES

Dental Disease

51 Smoking increases your risk of tooth decay.

Tooth decay starts with dental plaque, a film that forms on teeth from material in saliva. A cavity begins when certain bacteria in dental plaque work on sugars in your mouth to produce an acid that can dissolve tooth enamel and the dentin underneath the enamel. Brushing and flossing remove plaque, and a diet low in sugars can reduce decay.

Studies indicate that smokers have an increased risk of cavities in both the crowns and the roots of their teeth. Root cavities can occur when the gums recede due to periodontal disease (more common in smokers), exposing the tooth roots. If a cavity is not treated promptly, tooth pain, death of the tooth pulp, and a root abscess may ensue. Extraction of the tooth then might be necessary. Thus, smoking increases your risk of tooth loss from decay.

Exposure to secondhand smoke can also increase the risk of tooth decay. One study concluded that children exposed to secondhand smoke have double the risk of cavities compared to children not exposed.

52 Smokers have four times as much periodontal disease (gum disease) as nonsmokers and lose more teeth.

Periodontal disease involves deterioration of the gum tissue and the underlying bone in which the teeth are implanted. Periodontal disease begins with the interaction of sugars in foods with bacteria in the plaque that coats tooth surfaces. The resulting toxins can irritate gum tissue, causing bleeding and swelling. If you don't brush and floss away plaque regularly—and get periodic professional cleaning and scaling of your teeth—the plaque left on your teeth can harden into tartar, which further irritates your gums. Untreated, periodontal disease will cause the gum tissue to recede and the underlying bone to erode. The outcome is teeth that loosen and eventually fall out. Thus, periodontal disease, as well as tooth decay, causes tooth loss.

Periodontal disease may damage your health in other ways as well. Recent studies indicate that heart disease is more likely to occur in people with periodontal disease, because bacteria from diseased gums enter the bloodstream and damage the arteries. Stroke is also more likely to occur. Studies have also found that pregnant women who have severe periodontal disease are more likely to give birth to pre-term, low-birth-weight babies.

Smokers have four times as much periodontal disease as nonsmokers and tend to develop it at younger ages. And smokers' periodontal disease is usually more severe. The more you smoke, the worse your dental health is likely to be. Smokers are twice as likely to lose teeth as nonsmokers and are more likely to become toothless.

There are several reasons why smoking causes periodontal disease:

■ Tobacco smoke, as well as smokeless tobacco, is toxic to your gum tissues.

■ Smoking constricts the blood vessels in your gums so that fewer of the immune cells in your blood reach the sites of existing gum infection.

■ Smoking can reduce the number and activity of your immune cells.

■ Smokers often lack vitamin C in their systems, and a deficiency of this vitamin contributes to a breakdown in gum tissue.

■ Smokers are more likely than nonsmokers to habitually grind or clench their teeth, often during sleep, a condition called *bruxism*. Bruxism can erode teeth, gums, and the supporting bone.

■ Smoking increases the risk of osteoporosis, a disease that makes bones progressively more porous and fragile. Osteoporosis weakens the bone that holds your teeth in place.

If you continue to smoke while you are being treated for periodontal disease, the treatment is less likely to be successful than if you stopped. In smokers, the gums do not heal as quickly, antibacterial treatments are less successful, underlying bone treatments have poorer outcomes, and dental implants to replace missing teeth are more likely to fail.

On the other hand, if you quit smoking, over time your gums will likely regain healing abilities comparable to those of nonsmokers. And your risk of tooth loss will decrease.

Mouth Disease

53 **If a person with a common condition called *dry mouth* smokes, mouth infections are more likely.**

When your salivary glands produce too little saliva, the condition is called *dry mouth*. Millions of people have dry mouth. It is particularly common in the elderly. One study indicated that 24 percent of women and 18 percent of men have dry mouth. Sometimes, dry mouth is a temporary condition due to a salivary gland infection or blockage, a lack of vitamin C, or certain medicines. Over 200 medicines can cause dry mouth. If a medicine you take is causing dry mouth, it will, of course, help if you can stop taking that medicine—but this is not always an option.

Dry mouth can lead to difficulty swallowing, talking, and digesting food. You may develop abnormal taste or smell, burning of the mouth lining, tooth cavities, an inability to wear dentures, malnutrition, or infections of the tongue, mouth, or lips. Taking frequent sips of water, using an artificial saliva spray, and chewing sugarless candy all provide some relief.

If you have dry mouth, avoid smoking. Dry mouth makes your mouth tissues prone to infections, and tobacco smoke will irritate those tissues, making infections even more likely. In addition, smoking depletes your body of vitamin C. As noted above, a lack of vitamin C is one cause of dry mouth.

54 Smoking dulls your senses of taste and smell, which makes eating less enjoyable. A dull sense of taste or smell may jeopardize your health and safety.

Your senses of taste and smell are both involved in the enjoyment of food. Taste is the sensation experienced when taste buds on your tongue, and elsewhere in your mouth, detect substances dissolved in saliva. Your taste buds can detect five known sensations—sweet, bitter, sour, salty, and umami (savoriness)—but combinations of these sensations produce a wide spectrum of flavors.

Your nose, on the other hand, can detect and identify thousands of different odors—from gasoline to gardenias. Much of what we perceive as our sense of taste is really our sense of smell. Thus, when you eat a chocolate candy bar, you taste the sweetness of the sugar, but smell the aroma of the chocolate.

Acute senses of taste and smell provide a great many of life's pleasures. But an impaired sense of taste or smell may jeopardize health and safety for the following reasons:

- Some people with impaired taste or smell lose interest in food and undereat.

- Other people overeat in an attempt to find something that tastes good.

- Still others add unhealthy amounts of salt and sugar to food in an attempt to give food flavor.

- Someone who must limit salt intake, but is taste-impaired, may not be able to detect highly salted food.

- Smell-impaired people may omit vegetables from their diets because vegetables taste bitter to them.

- A person with an impaired sense of taste or smell may be unaware that food is spoiled, which could result in food poisoning.

- A person with an impaired sense of smell may be unable to detect the foul-smelling chemicals added to natural gas and propane to warn of gas leaks.

Aging, head injury, certain medicines, and various fumes can impair the senses of taste or smell. Smoking dulls both taste and smell. Moreover, smokers have more colds, flu, and sinus infections than nonsmokers. These can cause a temporary loss of the sense of smell.

When you quit smoking, both taste and smell ordinarily improve within a few days or weeks. The bad taste in your mouth goes away. Your sense of smell may take a longer time to recover than your sense of taste, but eventually it does. People who stop smoking are usually delighted with their renewed ability to taste and smell.

Throat Problems

55 Many smokers have chronic sore throats due to irritation from tobacco smoke, but find quick relief when they quit smoking.

Irritation from tobacco smoke can cause a persistent sore throat with discomfort or pain when swallowing. This condition is called *chronic pharyngitis* and ordinarily occurs in heavy smokers, but can occur in moderate smokers as well. If a chronically sore throat is accompanied by a cigarette cough, the cough further irritates the throat. Quitting—or at least cutting down on the number of cigarettes—usually relieves a smoker's sore throat.

But even if you think your sore throat is from smoking, see a doctor to make certain it is not a symptom of disease. A sore throat can be a symptom of many diseases, including streptococcus infection (strep throat), diphtheria, sinusitis, tonsillitis, syphilis, and throat cancer.

56 Smoking makes you more likely to suffer from laryngitis and hoarseness.

Most people suffer from *laryngitis*, an infection of the larynx (voice box), at one time or another, but smokers are more likely than nonsmokers to be affected. Laryngitis can cause hoarseness. Smokers sometimes develop chronic laryngitis and persistent hoarseness. There are a number of reasons why you are more likely to have laryngitis and hoarseness if you smoke.

First, laryngitis often follows a cold or flu. Smokers are more likely to get colds and flu than nonsmokers, and are therefore more apt to suffer from laryngitis and hoarseness. Moreover, smoking dries the throat and irritates the larynx, which can result in laryngitis, even in the absence of a cold or flu.

Second, backup of stomach acid into the larynx can irritate the vocal cords and cause hoarseness. Smoking may contribute to the buildup of stomach acid and is known to relax the sphincter at the juncture of the stomach and esophagus, allowing backup of stomach acid. Therefore, smokers are more likely than nonsmokers to suffer from hoarseness due to irritation of the vocal cords by stomach acid.

Third, smoking can cause polyps or ulcers on the vocal cords. A polyp is a benign growth, while an ulcer is a raw sore. Both polyps and ulcers result from misuse of the voice (yelling, loud speaking, or voice overuse) or inhalation of irritants such as tobacco smoke. A vocal cord polyp or ulcer can cause hoarseness, sometimes chronic hoarseness. A surgeon can remove a polyp to restore the patient's normal voice, but the patient must not smoke or more polyps will form. A patient with an ulcer on a vocal cord must quit smoking and rest the voice so that the ulcer can heal.

And, fourth, thickened white patches on the vocal cords, called *leukoplakia,* may cause hoarseness. Smoking is the most common cause of leukoplakia. Leukoplakia sometimes becomes cancerous. Quitting smoking may reverse tissue abnormalities in leukoplakia before they become cancerous.

Anyone who has been hoarse for more than two weeks should see a doctor. Chronic hoarseness is the most common symptom of cancer of the larynx. A smoker must be particularly vigilant because smokers have about ten times the risk of developing cancer of the larynx as people who have never smoked.

Diseases of the Esophagus, Stomach, and Intestines

57 **If you smoke you are more likely to get heartburn or *gastroesophageal reflux disease* (GERD), a serious illness that may result in esophageal cancer.**

Your esophagus is the muscular food tube leading directly into your stomach. At the juncture of your esophagus and stomach is a ring-like muscle, the *lower esophageal sphincter,* that normally opens to let food pass into the stomach, then closes to prevent food and stomach fluid from backing up into the esophagus. Your esophagus does not have your stomach's protective mucus coating to shield it from the irritating acids and enzymes in stomach fluid. So, if the sphincter opens when it shouldn't, stomach fluid can enter your esophagus, causing the burning sensation called heartburn.

Heartburn is a common malady that most people experience occasionally. However, frequent or constant heartburn may signal *gastroesophageal reflux disease* (GERD), also called "acid reflux." GERD is a serious illness that can cause scar tissue to form in the esophagus, narrowing it and leading to hoarseness and difficulty swallowing. Over time, GERD may result in esophageal cancer.

You can take a number of steps to prevent heartburn. It may help to avoid foods and beverages that trigger heartburn or make it worse—fatty, acidic, or spicy foods; peppermint; alcohol; and food or drinks that contain caffeine. If you stay up two to three hours after eating, and raise the head of your bed with six to eight inch blocks, this will help keep stomach contents where they belong. Losing excess weight and wearing loose clothing may help. And don't smoke. Smoking increases the likelihood of heartburn in three ways:

- Tobacco smoke contributes to the buildup of stomach acid.

- Smoking decreases the strength of your sphincter, allowing the backup of stomach acid into the esophagus.

■ The nicotine in tobacco smoke inhibits the production of saliva. Saliva acts as a buffer between your esophagus and stomach acid.

Clearly, if you suffer from frequent heartburn you should make every effort to quit smoking.

58 Smoking increases your risk of developing peptic ulcers, inhibits ulcer healing, and makes ulcers more likely to recur.

Ten percent of Americans have symptoms of peptic ulcer disease at some point in their lives, and twice as many show scarring from peptic ulcers on autopsy. A peptic ulcer is an open sore or erosion in the lining of the lower esophagus, the stomach, or the *duodenum* (the upper part of the small intestine where the stomach empties its contents). The duodenum is the most common site of peptic ulcers.

Symptoms that may alert you to peptic ulcers include a gnawing or burning pain in the upper abdomen (relieved by food or antacids); nausea; vomiting; or black, tarry stools that indicate bleeding. Untreated, peptic ulcers heal slowly and then recur in a large majority of cases. Treatment greatly reduces the risk of recurrence, and of complications such as persistent pain, uncontrolled bleeding, perforation of the stomach or intestine wall, and obstruction of the stomach/duodenal outlet due to scarring.

A number of factors contribute to the development of peptic ulcer disease, including infection with bacteria called *Helicobacter pylori*, regular use of aspirin and other nonsteroidal anti-inflammatory drugs (NSAIDs), an inherited tendency to peptic ulcer disease, and smoking. Not smoking is an important part of both the prevention and treatment of peptic ulcer disease. Smoking inhibits both spontaneous and medication-induced healing of ulcers. Furthermore, peptic ulcers are more likely to recur if you smoke. Because the tendency to develop peptic ulcers can be inherited, if you have a family history of the disease you should make a special effort to abstain from smoking.

59 Both current and former smokers have a four times greater risk of developing Crohn's disease than people who have never smoked.

Crohn's disease can affect any part of the digestive system, from the mouth to the lower colon. Most often it is a chronic inflammation of the intestinal wall that can cause pain and frequent diarrhea. One million Americans have Crohn's disease, including 100,000 children. The majority of cases start between the ages of 14 and 24, but new cases are not uncommon after age 50. Crohn's disease tends to run in families. Its cause is unknown. However, both current and former smokers have a four times greater risk of developing Crohn's disease than people who have never smoked.

Symptoms of Crohn's disease include diarrhea, abdominal cramps, fever, fatigue, bleeding, intestinal obstructions, intestinal abscesses, loss of appetite, malnutrition, and weight loss. Cancers of the colon and small intestine are more common in Crohn's patients than in the general population.

There is no known cure for Crohn's disease, but symptoms sometimes disappear for months or even years. The goal of treatment is to relieve the symptoms and prevent flare-ups with medication. In severe cases, damaged portions of the intestine are surgically removed. Smokers with Crohn's disease have significantly more flare-ups of symptoms. Doctors firmly counsel patients with Crohn's disease not to smoke.

EYE, EAR, AND SINUS DISEASES

Eye Diseases

60 **Smoking a pack of cigarettes a day doubles your risk of cataracts in your eyes. Heavier smoking increases your risk even more.**

The crystalline lens is a structure near the front of your eye that brings vision into focus. A normal lens is crystal clear. A *cataract* is a clouding of the lens that blocks the light needed for vision. Blurred vision and sensitivity to glare are symptoms of cataract. Ordinarily, both eyes are affected.

Cataracts are among the world's leading causes of blindness. Most people over age 60 have at least some lens clouding, although in many people the clouding does not progress to the point where surgery is necessary. Fortunately, surgery to remove the cloudy lens and replace it with a plastic implant lens is usually successful.

The cause of some cataracts isn't known, but it is known that cataracts are more common in people with eye inflammation, trauma to the eye, excessive alcohol consumption, diabetes, or excessive exposure to radiant energy (X-rays, microwaves, or strong sunlight). Smoking a pack of cigarettes a day doubles your risk of developing cataracts, and heavier smoking increases your risk even more. Moreover, in smokers, cataracts tend to develop at younger ages and to be more severe. And smokers are more likely to develop cataracts in the center of the lens, which impairs vision more than cataracts confined to the edges.

Experts advance several possible explanations as to why smoking promotes cataracts:

- Smoking reduces blood levels of certain vitamins that may help keep the crystalline lens transparent.

- Smoking can make arteriosclerosis worse and blood circulation poorer, which may reduce the nourishment available to the lens.

- Heavy metals such as cadmium in tobacco smoke may directly cause cataracts.

- Cigarette smoke constantly irritates the eyes, which may promote cataracts.

Quitting smoking lowers your risk of cataracts, although not to the level of people who have never smoked.

61 Age-related macular degeneration, the leading cause of permanent vision loss in people over age 60, is two to three times more common in smokers.

The *retina* is thin nerve tissue that lines the back of your eye and sends visual signals to your brain. The *macula* is the central area of your retina. The macula is responsible for clear, sharp central vision and for focusing on fine detail. The area of your retina that surrounds the macula is responsible for side, or peripheral, vision.

Deterioration of the macula in people over age 60 is called *age-related macular degeneration*. It is the leading cause of permanent central vision loss in older people. Middle-aged people have about a two percent risk of getting age-related macular degeneration. By age 75, almost 30 percent of people are affected to some degree, ranging from moderate visual impairment to legal blindness.

Macular degeneration usually affects both eyes. In many cases, there is no treatment, although in some cases new medications show promise. People who suffer a mild form of macular degeneration often benefit from using visual aids, such as magnifying devices, to enhance their central vision. People with severe macular degeneration become functionally blind.

Risk factors for developing macular degeneration include advancing age, light-colored eyes, a family history of the disease, and cigarette smoking. Studies show that if you smoke a pack or more a day, you have two to three times the risk of developing macular degeneration compared to people who have never smoked. The more cigarettes you smoke each day, and the more years you smoke, the greater your risk. Unfortunately, the risk does not seem to decrease significantly until you have stopped smoking for many years.

No one knows for certain why smoking increases your risk of age-related macular degeneration, but experts propose several logical hypotheses:

- The nicotine in tobacco smoke constricts blood vessels in the eyes, reducing their blood supply.

- Atherosclerosis is more common in smokers and narrows the arteries, including the arteries that supply blood to the eyes.

- Smoking lowers the body's level of certain antioxidant vitamins that protect the eyes.

- Smoking may cause a reduction in macular pigment that screens potentially harmful short-wave light.

Although the specific reasons why smoking increases your risk of macular degeneration may be uncertain, one thing is certain—you can avoid this increased risk by never smoking, or lessen it over time by quitting.

62 In people who have Graves' disease, a form of hyperthyroidism, smoking increases the risk of developing eye problems.

Hyperthyroidism is a disorder in which the thyroid gland, located in the base of your neck, produces too much *thyroxine*—a hormone necessary for many processes in the body. When there is too much thyroxine, body systems may function abnormally. Hyperthyroidism has been diagnosed in about a million Americans, mostly women between the ages of 20 and 40.

Graves' disease is by far the most common form of hyperthyroidism. People with Graves' disease often develop eye problems. The eyeballs may bulge forward from their sockets. The eyelids may not close completely, exposing the eyes to injury from dryness. The muscles that move the eyes may become swollen to the point that they are unable to function properly, resulting in double vision in many cases. In the most severe cases, the swollen muscles can exert pressure on the optic nerve sufficient to threaten vision, or even cause blindness.

Studies indicate that smokers with Graves' disease are at increased risk of developing eye problems. Such smokers also tend to have more severe eye problems than nonsmokers and may not respond as well to treatment. Smoking and Graves' disease are a bad combination.

Hearing Loss and Tinnitus

63 Smokers may be more likely to suffer hearing loss.

Hearing loss can be caused by aging, long-term exposure to excessive noise, ear infection or injury, or congenital defect. Hearing loss may be so gradual that you are unaware of it. Defective hearing can limit your ability to function in work, social, and recreational situations.

Although some studies have failed to establish smoking as a cause of hearing loss, other studies show that it is a cause. A study of 3,753 adults, aged 48 to 92, found that the smokers had a 70 percent higher rate of hearing loss than the nonsmokers.

Another study compared the hearing of 263 people, none of whom had been exposed to excessive noise. Compared to the nonsmokers under age 40:

- The smokers under age 40 had a 70 percent higher rate of hearing loss.

- The nonsmokers over age 40 had a 430 percent higher rate of hearing loss.

- The smokers over age 40 had a 750 percent higher rate of hearing loss.

The authors of this study concluded that the combination of aging and smoking is much more likely to cause hearing loss than either factor alone.

Exposure to loud noise and smoking are another combination that has been shown to be worse for your hearing than either factor alone. One study of steel workers exposed to noise on the job concluded that hearing loss among those who smoked was 156 percent higher than among nonsmoking employees not exposed to noise. Among the nonsmoking employees exposed to noise, hearing loss was 77 percent higher .

Some experts believe that cigarette smoke has a toxic effect on cells in your inner ear, causing hearing loss. Others believe that, because nicotine decreases the flow of blood to your hearing mechanism, over time a lack of oxygen and nourishment can cause hearing loss.

64 Smoking makes tinnitus worse.

An estimated 30 percent of older Americans suffer from *tinnitus*, or phantom noise. Tinnitus is noise that originates in your ear itself (some experts say in your brain), rather than in the environment. The noise may be a ringing, buzzing, hissing, roaring, tinkling, clanging, or whistling. Tinnitus may be mild and intermittent, or loud and constant. Some people are able to ignore or tolerate it. Others find that it seriously interferes with sleep and concentration, and results in great psychological distress.

Tinnitus is often associated with some degree of hearing loss, usually due to aging or long-term exposure to loud noises. Almost any ear disorder can cause tinnitus, as can migraine headaches, high blood pressure, arteriosclerosis, arthritis in the neck, thyroid disease, or injuries to the head or neck. Certain medications (aspirin, antibiotics, or antidepressants) sometimes trigger tinnitus. Excessive caffeine or alcohol consumption, and smoking may also contribute to the development of tinnitus.

A device that is worn in the ear and produces pleasant sounds may help mask the noise, but tinnitus is usually impossible to cure. Tobacco smoke, like other stimulants, makes tinnitus worse. If you are a smoker with tinnitus you may gain some relief by quitting.

Sinusitis

65 You will be less likely to get sinusitis if you don't smoke and if you avoid exposure to secondhand smoke.

Sinusitis is a common affliction, affecting millions of Americans. Your sinuses are hollow air spaces in the bone structure around your eyes and nose. Your sinuses are lined with mucus membranes and open into your nose, so anything that causes swelling in your nose—such as a cold or an allergy attack—can swell your sinus membranes, narrowing or closing off the sinus openings.

Reduced or blocked drainage of mucus from your sinuses can lead to infection with bacteria—that is, to *acute bacterial sinusitis*. Acute bacterial sinusitis usually causes sinus tenderness or pain, and sometimes fever. Repeated bouts of acute bacterial sinusitis, especially if they are not properly treated with antibiotics, can lead to *chronic sinusitis*. In rare cases, sinusitis causes an infection of the facial bones, or of the membranes enclosing the brain (*meningitis*).

Smokers are especially vulnerable to sinusitis for two reasons. First, colds often precede sinusitis and smokers get more colds than nonsmokers. Second, tobacco smoke irritates your sinus membranes, which can cause sinusitis.

Therefore, you will be less likely to get sinusitis if you don't smoke and if you avoid exposure to secondhand smoke.

BONE DISEASE AND BACK PAIN

Osteoporosis

66 **Smoking increases your risk of osteoporosis, a bone condition that can result in severe back pain, deformity, disability, and death.**

The density of your bones increases from childhood until about age 35, then slowly begins to decrease, making the bones progressively more porous and fragile. Low bone density (*osteopenia*) is extremely common, affecting about 40 percent of American women over age 50 and 33 percent of men over age 70. Full-blown *osteoporosis* is severe bone loss, meaning that the bones have become so porous and fragile that they fracture easily. One study showed that women with osteopenia were about twice as likely as women with normal bones to suffer a fracture. Women with osteoporosis were four times as likely.

Your bones derive their hardness from calcium. The female hormone estrogen or the male hormone testosterone are necessary to absorb calcium from the diet and keep bones dense. Unless they undergo hormone replacement therapy, women lose bone density rapidly after menopause when their ovaries are no longer producing estrogen. Testosterone production in men declines only gradually with age, so until age 65 to 70 men lose bone density more slowly. Because men have larger bones to begin with, and lose bone density more slowly, fewer men than women develop osteoporosis. But once men reach age 65 to 70 they begin to lose bone density at the same rate as women. One third of hip fractures occur in men.

Osteoporosis is a "silent disease"—that is, you are unaware that it is happening. Bone density screening, beginning about age 50 for women and later for men, can enable you to start preventive therapy before you have lost a significant amount of bone and are at risk for fractures. There are a number of drugs that can increase your bone density.

Unfortunately, in many people the first symptom of osteoporosis is a bone fracture, usually in the wrist, hip, or spine. A wrist or hip bone may break upon minor impact, such as lifting a bag of groceries or stepping off a curb. The vertebrae may fracture and compress, causing severe back pain, a gradual loss of height, and a deformed backbone that curves forward (a "dowager's hump").

About 20 percent of people with hip fractures die of complications within a year. Many people with hip fractures suffer permanent disability. Fractures heal slowly in people with osteoporosis. More than half of those who survive a broken hip need long-term care in a nursing facility or at home. Wrist fractures cause temporary disability by making dressing, housekeeping, shopping and other activities difficult or impossible. Back pain from fractures of the vertebrae also can cause disability.

Prevention of osteoporosis is extremely important. Prevention should begin early in life with the following regimen that builds up the maximum amount of bone:

■ Good nutrition from a diet with sufficient calcium.

■ Sufficient vitamin D, which is essential to calcium absorption.

■ Regular weight-bearing exercise, which stimulates bone formation.

Prevention of osteoporosis also includes avoidance of the following:

■ Excessive alcohol consumption, which reduces bone formation.

■ Cigarette smoking and secondhand smoke, both of which decrease bone density.

Researchers estimate that six to ten percent of hip fractures are attributable to smoking. Smoking decreases your bone density and increases the risk of osteoporosis and fracture in a number of ways. First, smoking reduces the blood supply to your bones, slows the production of bone-forming cells, and impairs the absorption of calcium. Second, because of all the health problems caused by smoking—poor lung function, angina, heart disease, and emphysema, among others—smokers are less likely to engage in the regular weight-bearing exercise (walking, jogging, or running) that stimulates bone formation. Third, smokers are more likely than nonsmokers to be underweight. Underweight people are at greater risk of developing osteoporosis than people who are heavier.

Finally, smoking interferes with the production of testosterone in men and estrogen in women. And women who smoke enter menopause about two years sooner than nonsmokers. Hormone replacement therapy (HRT) replaces estrogen and is an effective method of curbing bone loss, but is not recommended for a woman who smokes.

What's more, studies indicate that smoking negates HRT's beneficial effect on the bones.

Broken Bones

67 Smoking slows the healing of broken bones.

Normal, healthy bones can be broken by a sudden, severe impact. Falls, sports injuries, and automobile accidents are common causes of broken bones. Bones that have become porous and fragile because of osteoporosis may break as the result of a minor impact.

Ordinarily, a bone fracture is treated by a physician as soon as X-rays or other tests indicate the nature of the break. A bone fracture often requires realigning broken pieces and securing them with a cast, brace, or splint. Sometimes a metal plate or rod is attached internally to the pieces of broken bone. Fracture treatment immobilizes the bone so that it can heal properly, but prolonged immobilization weakens the bone and the surrounding muscle. The sooner the bone heals and the sooner normal use of the bone and muscle can be resumed, the better.

Smoking slows the healing of broken bones. One study showed that broken legs healed 80 percent faster in nonsmokers than in smokers. Therefore, a smoker's broken bone must be immobilized longer. This increases weakening of the bone and surrounding muscle, lengthens the period of disability, and prolongs pain.

Experts believe that smokers' bones heal more slowly because cigarette smoke impedes blood circulation, causing less oxygen to reach the cells that produce substances necessary to patch the bone. In smokers with bone fractures due to osteoporosis, healing may be slower yet because porous, fragile bones heal more slowly than normal bones. Abstaining from smoking can shorten the time a broken bone will take to heal.

Back Pain

68 Smoking increases your risk of back pain and sciatica.

The upright posture of humans depends on a strong, flexible column of backbones linked by ligaments and supported by muscles in the back and abdomen. Exercises that promote a healthy back by strengthening these muscles include walking, cycling, and swimming. In addition, there are exercises specifically designed to strengthen muscles that support the back. Studies show that smokers are less likely than nonsmokers to engage in regular exercise, and therefore are less likely to have strong muscles for back support.

Back pain is an extremely common ailment. About 80 percent of the population will have back pain at some time in their lives. Moreover, back pain tends to recur. Causes of back pain include muscle strains and spasms, sprained ligaments, ruptured disks, osteoporosis, spinal arthritis, cancer, and aortic aneurysms.

The most common cause of back pain is a small tear within the back muscles, called a strain. Straining your back muscles sends them into spasm (involuntary contractions), which causes pain and limits movement. Back ligaments are also subject to injuries, called sprains. The nicotine in cigarettes constricts your blood vessels and decreases blood supply to an injured muscle or ligament, thus healing is slower and back pain lasts longer. Moreover, a cigarette cough can be extremely irritating to your back muscles, sending them into spasm.

A less common cause of back pain is a *herniated spinal disk,* often called a "ruptured disk." Your spinal disks act as cushions between each pair of vertebrae. Spinal disks have a tough, fibrous outer cover enclosing jellylike inner material. If the outer cover becomes weakened, the disk may rupture and the jellylike material protrude and press upon a nerve, causing pain or numbness. Disk pressure on the sciatic nerve—the nerve that begins in your lower back and branches down the length of each leg—results in sciatic pain (sciatica) in the buttock and back of the leg. Trauma or aging can weaken the fibrous outer cover of the spinal disks, and an increasing number of studies indicate that smoking also causes disk degeneration. Moreover, a chronic cigarette cough increases pain from ruptured disks.

Older people may have back pain as a result of osteoporosis, a condition in which the bones have become so porous and fragile that they fracture easily. In a person with osteoporosis the bones of the spine are among those most prone to fracture. Even everyday activities such as lifting a bag of groceries or raising a window can trigger tiny fractures in the spine. If the bones in the spine fracture and compress, severe back pain can result. Although spinal fractures mend, pain sometimes lingers for months. Smoking decreases your bone density and increases your risk of osteoporosis, so you are at greater risk of back pain from spinal fractures if you smoke.

Arthritic changes in the spine sometimes result in back pain, especially in people over age 50. Exercise is one of the best long-term strategies to combat back pain caused by spinal arthritis. However, because of other health problems caused by smoking, older smokers may be unable to do the exercise that helps this type of back pain.

Cancer affecting the bones in the spine is yet another cause of back pain. Most bone cancers have metastasized from another location. Lung and kidney cancers are among the most likely to spread to bone. Smoking causes the great majority of lung cancers and is the most important risk factor for kidney cancer. Therefore, smokers are more likely than nonsmokers to suffer back pain from cancer that has spread to the spine.

An aortic aneurysm also can cause back pain, sometimes severe back pain. An aortic aneurysm is a bulge, or weakened area, in the aorta—the major artery in your chest and abdomen. Smoking weakens your blood vessels and greatly increases the risk of aortic aneurysm.

AUTOIMMUNE DISEASES

Lupus

69 **Smoking may increase the risk of lupus, makes the effects of lupus worse, and interferes with the treatment of lupus.**

Systemic lupus erythematosus—called, simply, "lupus"—is a chronic disease causing inflammation of the connective tissues. The connective tissues are essential elements of every part of your body. Lupus is an *autoimmune disease*, that is, a disease in which the immune system attacks the body's own tissues, mistaking them for foreign invaders such as bacteria, viruses, or fungi.

An estimated one million Americans have lupus. It tends to run in families and primarily affects young women, although men, children, and older people do get it. African Americans, Hispanics, Native Americans, and some Asian Americans are more likely than Caucasians to contract lupus.

Lupus symptoms include fever, rashes, a sick feeling, loss of appetite, weight loss, joint pain, and problems with lung, kidney, and heart function. Lupus may also cause hair loss and scarring of the skin that can be devastating to patients. Symptoms may flare up and then subside on their own. Because early symptoms are often vague or easily confused with symptoms of other diseases, lupus may not be diagnosed for years. It is a disease that can be mild, but is more often severe, sometimes even life-threatening. A number of studies indicate that smoking may increase your risk of developing lupus, especially if you have a genetic tendency toward the disease.

Moreover, smoking makes the effects of lupus worse. For example, people with lupus are susceptible to pneumonia, and smokers with lupus are especially susceptible. Lupus can also cause narrowing of the blood vessels and increase the risk of blood clots. Smoking compounds these effects of lupus. Kidney disease may develop in people with lupus. If they smoke they will progress to end-stage kidney disease far more quickly.

Lupus is incurable, but medications can treat many cases effectively. However, smoking interferes with the action of antimalarial drugs used to treat skin disease caused by lupus. Other medications used to treat lupus increase the risk of osteoporosis. Smoking also increases the risk of osteoporosis and makes it even more likely that the lupus patient will develop fragile bones. Experts say that quitting cigarettes is the most important lifestyle change that you can make if you have lupus.

Rheumatoid Arthritis

70 Smoking can increase your susceptibility to rheumatoid arthritis and increase the disease's severity.

Rheumatoid arthritis is an *autoimmune disease*—that is, a disease in which the immune system attacks parts of the body. Rheumatoid arthritis affects the connective tissues. Joints become inflamed, resulting in swelling, stiffness, and pain. Deterioration and deformity of the joints may occur.

About one to two percent of Americans are afflicted with rheumatoid arthritis—three times as many women as men. Onset of the disease is usually between 20 and 50 years, but it can begin at any age. Untreated, rheumatoid arthritis can damage the heart, lungs, nerves, or eyes.

The exact cause of rheumatoid arthritis is unknown, although people who have family members with the disease are more prone to develop it. And a number of studies demonstrate that smoking increases your susceptibility to rheumatoid arthritis. Other studies indicate that smoking can make rheumatoid arthritis more severe. Anyone with a family history of rheumatoid arthritis, and certainly those who already have developed the disease, should avoid smoking.

Raynaud's Disease

71 **If you have Raynaud's disease, smoking makes attacks of the disease more likely and more severe.**

About one in 20 Americans, mostly women, suffer from Raynaud's disease. Raynaud's disease is an exaggeration of the body's normal response to cold, in which blood vessels constrict, particularly in the extremities. In Raynaud's disease, the blood vessels in the fingers (the site usually affected) or toes virtually clamp shut. Fingers or toes turn white, then blue, and finally red. An attack causes numbness, tingling, burning, and sometimes pain, and can last for minutes or hours. Applying warmth usually restores normal color and sensation. But sometimes there is irreversible tissue injury.

Ordinarily, these attacks occur when someone with Raynaud's disease is exposed to cold, is under stress, or smokes cigarettes. Smoking clogs and constricts blood vessels, making Raynaud's attacks more likely and more severe. And smoking may have a role in the irreversible tissue injury that sometimes occurs in people with Raynaud's disease. Anyone who has Raynaud's disease needs medical attention, because in some cases Raynaud's disease is a symptom of another disease that is more serious, particularly the autoimmune disease scleroderma, and sometimes lupus or rheumatoid arthritis.

WOUNDS AND SURGERY

Wounds

72 **Smokers have more wound infections, slower healing wounds, and larger scars from wounds than nonsmokers.**

Injuries to the skin and underlying tissue range from minor scratches to life-threatening wounds. People ordinarily deal with minor wounds themselves. More serious wounds require medical treatment.

Despite proper treatment, any wound can become infected—even a surgical incision. Infection can spread to adjacent organs, or be carried to distant areas of the body through the blood. Infection delays wound healing and may result in disability, or even death. Those most susceptible to wound infection are people with certain illnesses (AIDS, diabetes, or cancer), the obese, the elderly, and smokers.

In addition to being more susceptible to wound infection, if you smoke you are more likely to have slow-healing wounds. Smoking reduces the number of certain cells necessary for wound repair. The oxygen that is also necessary for wound repair is diminished by the carbon monoxide in tobacco smoke. The blood carries substances necessary for wound repair to the wound site. Nicotine in tobacco smoke constricts blood vessels so that less blood flows to the wound site.

Studies have linked smoking with slow healing of various types of wounds. For example, one study found that smoking slows the healing of bedsores (pressure ulcers). Smoking decreases the healing rate after surgical removal of impacted teeth. Rupture of abdominal incisions occurs more often in smokers than in nonsmokers. Smokers' skin grafts are more likely to fail. In cosmetic surgery, including facelifts, breast lifts, and tummy tucks, the skin is separated from underlying tissues, creating a "flap." Smoking increases the chance that the skin flap will die, creating a more unsightly problem than was there at the start. But if you refrain from smoking before and after you have any surgery, you can improve your chances of a successful outcome. And if you don't smoke after receiving a wound caused by trauma, the wound will heal faster.

Slow-healing wounds result in larger scars. Studies have shown that smokers are likely to develop larger scars than nonsmokers with comparable wounds. Plastic surgeons are sometimes able to "revise" scars to make them smaller and less noticeable. In a scar revision, the scar is cut out and the incision re-closed. But if you smoke you will not be a good candidate to have an unattractive scar revised.

Surgery

73 **If you smoke you are more likely than a nonsmoker to need certain types of surgery, to have complications from surgery, and to have a poorer long-term outcome after surgery.**

Smokers are at a serious disadvantage compared to nonsmokers in regard to surgery. First, smokers are more likely than nonsmokers to have disorders that may make surgery necessary—including heart and blood vessel disease, cancer, emphysema, collapsed lung, cataracts, gum disease, Crohn's disease, and hip fractures.

Second, smokers are more likely to have complications under general anesthesia. General anesthesia is often necessary for major surgery. It puts the patient to sleep and slows the heartbeat, breathing, and other vital functions. Smokers are usually more difficult to anesthetize than nonsmokers, and have an increased risk of breathing problems, and even death, when under general anesthesia.

Third, long-term smoking increases the likelihood of chronic obstructive pulmonary disease (COPD), coronary artery disease, and heart failure. COPD increases the risk of respiratory problems during general anesthesia. Coronary artery disease makes the risk of heart attack during major surgery at least four times as likely. A patient with heart failure who undergoes major surgery has a two to ten percent risk of cardiac arrest during the procedure.

Fourth, after surgery, smokers are at greater risk for respiratory problems—six times greater, according to one study. Smokers and people with COPD (nearly always caused by smoking) are at increased risk for pneumonia. Smokers are also at increased risk of broncospasm, a condition that causes partial obstruction of the airways. They are more likely to need supplemental oxygen, or a prolonged period on a mechanical breathing apparatus.

Fifth, smokers have a greater risk of infection in their surgical incisions, and their incisions are more likely to burst open or to heal slowly. Furthermore, surgical incisions in smokers result in larger scars than those in nonsmokers.

And, sixth, studies show that the long-term outcome of many types of surgery is less favorable in smokers. Here are a few examples:

- Bypass surgery to circumvent clogged blood vessels in the legs is twice as likely to fail in smokers.

- Long-term survival rates are significantly reduced in smokers undergoing coronary artery bypass surgery, and in heart transplant patients who continue to smoke after transplantation.

- Surgical removal of the lining of a clogged carotid artery (the artery in the neck that supplies blood to the brain) is more likely to have to be repeated if the patient is a smoker.

- Replantation of a smoker's severed finger is more likely to fail.

- A smoker's cosmetic surgery is less likely to be successful.

Physicians often urge smokers to abstain from tobacco for at least eight weeks before major surgery. This smoke-free period eliminates carbon monoxide from the blood, reduces mucus production in the lungs, improves the action of the cilia that sweep the airways free of mucus and debris, and strengthens the immune system.

But much major surgery is done on an emergency basis, in which case the smoker will not have an opportunity to stop smoking eight weeks before surgery. And abstaining for eight weeks will not reverse conditions common in smokers that increase the risks of surgery—COPD, coronary artery disease, and heart failure, among others.

SLEEP PROBLEMS

Insomnia

74 If you smoke you are more likely to suffer from chronic insomnia.

Almost everyone occasionally experiences a sleepless night or two, but *chronic insomnia* affects an estimated 15 to 20 percent of adults. Chronic insomnia is defined as a month or more of difficulty falling asleep or staying asleep. Chronic insomniacs have more illnesses and recover from illnesses more slowly. Lack of sleep depresses your immune system, making it less effective in defending against disease-causing microorganisms and cancer cells. One study indicated that getting enough sleep may be nearly as important to the health of your heart as a good diet and enough exercise. Another study reported that adults who sleep six hours or less a night have significantly higher death rates from all causes than those who sleep seven or eight hours.

Chronic insomnia also reduces your alertness, thereby increasing the dangers of driving and operating machinery. Some research data show that a drowsy automobile driver may be as likely to crash as a drunk driver. Drowsy drivers cause an estimated 100,000 automobile crashes a year. And sleep deprivation can result in injuries and deaths on the job, especially when a drowsy person flies an airplane, operates heavy machinery, or drives a truck, bus, or train. In addition to the risk of accidents, too little sleep makes you irritable, and adversely affects your memory, attention, concentration, creativity, and ability to make decisions.

Some people get relief from insomnia by engaging in regular aerobic exercise (although not right before bedtime), reducing stress, going to bed and getting up at regular times, sleeping in a quiet, comfortable, cool, dark room, and avoiding alcohol (that can cause light, fitful sleep), caffeine, and tobacco. Compared to nonsmokers, smokers are more likely to suffer from chronic insomnia for several reasons:

■ The nicotine in cigarettes is a powerful stimulant that may prevent the smoker from going to sleep.

■ Nicotine withdrawal may cause craving for a cigarette that awakens the smoker in the middle of the night. Smoking a cigarette to quell the craving makes it difficult to go back to sleep because of nicotine's stimulant effect.

■ Smokers are more likely to suffer from conditions that interfere with sleep, including angina (heart pain), chronic cough, shortness of breath, sinusitis, heartburn, chronic bronchitis, emphysema, congestive heart failure, peptic ulcers, anxiety, depression, snoring, and sleep apnea.

Sleep quality matters as much as quantity. A normal sleep cycle includes a progression from drowsiness to moderate sleep to deep restorative sleep, as well as four or five periods of "rapid-eye-movement sleep" when most dreaming occurs. Heavy smokers experience less deep sleep and less rapid-eye-movement sleep. After people quit smoking, they tend to fall asleep more quickly and sleep more soundly than they did when they smoked, although their sleep may be disrupted temporarily during the quitting process.

Snoring

75 Smokers are more likely than nonsmokers to be habitual snorers.

Snoring occurs during sleep when air rushing through the mouth vibrates soft tissue in the back of the throat (the soft palate). Although most people snore occasionally, an habitual snorer is most likely to be an overweight, middle-aged man who smokes. Partial obstruction of the breathing passages—due to relaxation of the muscles at the back of the throat, or to nasal blockage—causes snoring. Smoking can inflame your nasal passages and swell your throat tissues, increasing the obstruction that causes snoring.

You may be unaware that you snore. But your snoring may disrupt the sleep of a spouse or roommate, who will most likely tell you. Corrective surgery or injections into the soft palate are used to treat extreme cases of snoring. However, most snorers improve when they lose weight, avoid alcohol and sedatives (both of which relax muscles in the back of the throat), and stop smoking.

Sleep Apnea

76 If you smoke, especially if you smoke heavily, you are at much greater risk of developing sleep apnea than nonsmokers or former smokers.

Someone with *sleep apnea* repeatedly stops breathing during sleep when the airway muscles collapse, temporarily blocking the airway. Arousing slightly in a struggle to resume breathing, the person with sleep apnea may snore loudly as breathing resumes. Many people with sleep apnea do not remember these arousals, which can happen hundreds of times a night. They are tired and sleepy in the daytime, but may not know why. Although most snorers do not have sleep apnea, if you are a snorer who is tired and sleepy during the day, tell your doctor. Doctors advise snorers who suffer from daytime fatigue and sleepiness to undergo an overnight sleep study to determine if they have sleep apnea.

Sleep apnea is a dangerous disorder that requires medical treatment. People with sleep apnea suffer from oxygen deprivation and are at increased risk of high blood pressure, heart disease, and stroke. They are prone to automobile crashes and other accidents. One study showed that people with sleep apnea have seven times as many automobile crashes as people without it. They may be unable to concentrate, have impaired memory and judgment, and be irritable and depressed. Job loss and family problems can result. Men suffering from sleep apnea may experience sexual dysfunction.

Sleep apnea affects nine percent of men and four percent of women over age 30. The typical man with sleep apnea is overweight, with a short, thick neck. The typical woman is obese. Sleep apnea seems to run in families.

If you smoke, especially if you smoke heavily, you are at much greater risk of developing sleep apnea than a nonsmoker or former smoker. One study indicated that people who smoke more than 40 cigarettes a day are four times more likely to have sleep apnea than nonsmokers. Sleep apnea, like snoring, may improve if the person loses weight, avoids alcohol and sedatives, and quits smoking. If these measures are not enough, medical and surgical options can control sleep apnea.

SEXUAL AND HORMONAL PROBLEMS

Impotence

77 **Smoking increases a man's risk of becoming impotent.**

Many men have a nagging fear of losing the ability to achieve and maintain an erection sufficient for sexual intercourse. An erection occurs when the arteries in the penis widen and the veins narrow. Blood then rushes into the penis and becomes trapped, producing an erection.

Every man has occasional difficulty getting or maintaining an erection, but when the problem is frequent or chronic, the condition is called *erectile dysfunction*, or impotence. About five percent of American men are impotent by age 40, and 33 percent over age 60 are impotent. Impotence can put a strain on marriage and other intimate relationships.

Some cases of impotence are due to psychological causes or the side effects of certain medications (tranquilizers, antidepressants, anti-inflammatory drugs, and blood pressure medications). However, the majority of cases, about 75 percent, can be traced to underlying physical conditions. Atherosclerosis (plaque deposits in artery walls) is one of the most common, affecting the arteries in the penis so that they don't expand as much, or become blocked. Smoking is a major risk factor for atherosclerosis. Men can reduce the risk of impotence with a regimen to prevent atherosclerosis—

that is, a healthy diet, regular exercise, medication in some cases, and not smoking.

Men who smoke are much more likely to become impotent, and young men, as well as the elderly, are at risk. A federal government study showed that, in a large group of men 31 to 49 years of age, the rate of impotence among the smokers was 50 percent higher than among the nonsmokers. Moreover, the drug Viagra is less effective in combating smokers' impotence because smokers' damaged blood vessels are less responsive to the drug. Fortunately, there is evidence that quitting smoking may improve erectile function.

Menstrual Pain

78 Smoking increases the occurrence, severity, and duration of menstrual pain.

Menstrual pain, often called "cramps," is one of the most common complaints of women during the years of menstruation. Menstrual pain affects young women more often than older women. About 50 to 75 percent of women experience this problem at some time in their lives. About five to six percent of women suffer pain severe enough to interfere with normal activities. This makes menstrual pain a leading cause of absence from school and work among menstrual-aged women—causing an estimated 140 million lost work hours in the United States each year.

Certain diseases, including *endometriosis* (a condition in which fragments of uterine lining are found in other parts of the pelvic cavity), fibroid tumors in the uterus, pelvic inflammatory disease, or malposition of the uterus, can cause menstrual pain, especially in older women. So it is important to have a doctor rule out disease as the cause of menstrual pain. But most menstrual pain results from contractions of the uterus and constriction of uterine blood vessels, causing a lack of oxygen to the uterus.

Nonsteroidal anti-inflammatory drugs (NSAIDS), such as aspirin, ibuprofen, or naproxen, are often helpful in treating menstrual pain. Heat applied to the abdomen or back, or hot baths, may provide some relief. Oral contraceptives (birth control pills) are effective in treating menstrual pain, because they prevent ovulation (the monthly release of an egg from an ovary). Where there is no underlying disease, menstrual pain does not occur without ovulation.

Studies in the United States and Europe show that smoking increases the occurrence, severity, and duration of menstrual pain. The risk of menstrual pain rises as the quantity of cigarettes smoked rises. What's more, a smoker may be precluded from taking oral contraceptives to treat menstrual pain because the combination of smoking and oral contraceptives increases the risk of heart attack, stroke, and deep vein thrombosis.

Birth Control

79 The combination of smoking and taking birth control pills increases your risk of heart attack, stroke, and deep vein thrombosis.

Used correctly, birth control pills offer almost 100 percent protection against pregnancy. Birth control pills also have these other advantages:

■ Their protection against pregnancy is reversible—
that is, if you stop taking them you regain your ability
to become pregnant.

■ They result in lighter, more regular menstrual
periods, and relieve menstrual cramps.

■ They protect against cancers of the ovaries and
uterine lining—protection that lasts long after you
stop taking birth control pills.

■ They decrease the risk of pelvic inflammatory
disease, fibrocystic breast disease, fibroid tumors of
the uterus, and benign ovarian cysts.

■ They improve bone density.

■ They are an effective treatment for acne.

Some of these same advantages apply also to the newer
hormone-based birth control methods, including the
Mirena IUD, NuvaRing, Implanon, Depo-subQ Provera
104, Seasonique, and Lybrel. Despite these advantages of
birth control pills and the newer hormone-based birth
control methods, doctors often advise smokers, especially
heavy smokers and smokers over age 35, not to use them. A
smoker who uses hormone-based birth control has an
increased risk of heart attack, stroke, and deep vein
thrombosis.

80 Women who smoke heavily, and even light smokers over age 35, are not candidates to take the abortion pill.

Mifepristone (RU-486), a prescription medicine popularly
called the "abortion pill", was developed in France and has
been used there since 1988. Other European countries

followed suit in the 1990s. The abortion pill was approved for use in the United States in September 2000. It offers an alternative to surgical abortion, an alternative that is appealing to many women.

In France in 1991, after a 31-year-old woman who smoked heavily suffered a heart attack while attempting to abort her thirteenth pregnancy with the abortion pill, the French government banned use of the pill by heavy smokers. In the United States, doctors do not prescribe the abortion pill for women who smoke heavily because there are no clinical data on its safety in heavy smokers. The same is true of women over 35 who smoke ten or more cigarettes per day, because they were generally excluded from clinical trials of the pill.

Menopause and Hormone Replacement Therapy

81 Menopause begins one to two years earlier in women who smoke.

Menopause is the permanent cessation of menstruation. Menopause usually occurs between 45 and 55 years of age, 51 being average. As a woman approaches menopause, her estrogen production declines. About 85 percent of women have unpleasant physical or emotional problems at this time. Of even greater concern is the increased risk of heart disease and the loss of bone mass that occur when estrogen declines.

In women who smoke, menopause begins one to two years earlier than in nonsmokers. And, if you are a woman who smokes, the more you smoke the earlier your menopause is likely to begin. Fortunately, this effect may be wholly or partly reversible if you stop smoking well before menopause. One study of menopausal women who had stopped smoking before age 35 showed that they began menopause only about 2.5 months earlier than women who had never smoked.

82 Hormone replacement therapy is not recommended if you are a woman who smokes.

Female hormones govern a woman's menstrual cycle. Menstruation ceases at an average age of 51 because the hormone estrogen secreted by the ovaries declines with age. Sometimes menstruation ceases earlier because the woman's ovaries have been surgically removed.

The lack of estrogen after the permanent cessation of menstruation (menopause) can create a number of physical and emotional problems. To combat some of these problems, physicians may prescribe estrogen in pills or a skin patch. A woman who has not had her uterus (womb) removed also takes progestin to help prevent uterine cancer. The combination of estrogen and progestin therapy is called *hormone replacement therapy* (HRT). HRT has definite risks and benefits. Its use must be carefully tailored to the needs of each woman.

HRT combats the post-menopausal loss of bone mass that may result in osteoporosis (thinning of the bones) and bone fractures. Other benefits of HRT include relief from hot flashes and night sweats, reduction of insomnia, and maintenance of pre-menopausal levels of vaginal lubrication, so that sexual intercourse is comfortable. Research indicates that estrogen therapy provides some protection against colon cancer, but may increase the risk of breast cancer.

Because the combination of smoking and HRT increases the risk of heart attack, stroke, and deep vein thrombosis (blood clots in the legs that can migrate to the lungs and may cause death), HRT is not recommended if you are a woman who smokes. But if you stop smoking, you may be able to undergo HRT.

REPRODUCTION PROBLEMS

Infertility

83 **Smoking contributes to infertility in women and, to a lesser extent, in men.**

A complex chain of events takes place before a pregnancy occurs—development of an egg in the woman's ovary, the egg's expulsion from the ovary, its journey down the fallopian tube (the tube that connects the ovary to the uterus), its fertilization by a man's sperm, and its implantation in the woman's uterus. Hormones control this process. A problem at any stage of the process can result in infertility.

Infertility is increasingly common in the United States, largely because people now marry when they are older and wait longer to have children. Both men and women are most fertile in their teens and twenties. A couple is said to be infertile if the woman does not become pregnant after a year of normal sexual intercourse without birth control. Infertility affects 15 to 20 percent of couples. About 60 percent of couples who have been unsuccessful in achieving pregnancy after a year of trying eventually do achieve pregnancy, either with or without medical intervention.

Only the woman is infertile in 50 percent of infertility cases and only the man is infertile in 30 percent. Both are infertile in 20 percent of cases. Major causes of infertility include problems with ovulation (the release of an egg), with the woman's fallopian tubes, with her uterus, or with the man's sperm.

Smoking contributes to infertility in women and, to a lesser extent, in men. Women who smoke are more apt to suffer from pelvic inflammatory disease that may cause blockages in the fallopian tubes, where conception usually occurs. Such blockages interfere with the passage of the woman's eggs and the man's sperm through the fallopian tubes.

Even without one of these problems, a woman who smokes reduces her chance of becoming pregnant. Some studies point to an adverse effect on the hormones that govern reproduction. Other studies have found that smoking lowers the rate of entry of eggs into the fallopian tube, or reduces the beating of the cilia (hairlike projections in the fallopian tube that propel the egg toward the uterus). Some studies indicate that smoking may damage the eggs themselves

Whatever the reasons, many studies have demonstrated a reduced likelihood of pregnancy in women who smoke. Even light smokers may have reduced fertility. A woman who is trying to become pregnant should stop smoking, not only to increase her chance of conceiving, but also to prevent the harm that smoking can do to her baby if she does conceive.

The effects of smoking on fertility in men are less clear. A few studies have shown no association between a man's smoking and his fertility. Other studies have demonstrated that men who smoke are more likely to have poor semen quality, with a greater number of abnormal sperm, a low sperm count, or sperm that have less mobility. Semen quality may improve if the man quits smoking. Higher semen quality increases the likelihood of pregnancy. In addition, a man who smokes is more likely to suffer from impotence (the inability to maintain an erection), which is an obstacle to making his partner pregnant.

Ectopic Pregnancy

84 **Smoking more than doubles a woman's risk of ectopic pregnancy. Ectopic pregnancy may result in a medical emergency requiring removal of a fallopian tube. Removal of a fallopian tube cuts in half the woman's chance of becoming pregnant.**

A woman has two fallopian tubes, one leading from each ovary to the uterus. During each menstrual cycle, an egg is released from one ovary and travels down its fallopian tube toward the uterus, being swept along by tiny hairlike projections called cilia. If sperm are present, they swim up the fallopian tube to meet the egg. Fertilization of the egg normally takes place in the fallopian tube.

In a normal pregnancy, the fertilized egg travels down the fallopian tube and implants itself in the lining of the uterus, where it begins to develop. However, in about one in every 100 pregnancies the fertilized egg implants itself in an abnormal site, usually in the fallopian tube, but occasionally in an ovary or other site. This is called an *ectopic pregnancy* (or a *tubal pregnancy* when the egg implants itself in a fallopian tube). Early signs of ectopic pregnancy include menstrual delay followed by vaginal bleeding, and abdominal pain that may become severe.

Sometimes the body releases the developing egg and the embryo is aborted (miscarried). If the embryo is not aborted and if the ectopic pregnancy is diagnosed soon enough, a surgeon can remove the embryo from the fallopian tube before the growth of the embryo causes the tube to rupture. Rupture of a fallopian tube causes intense pain and bleeding. It is a medical emergency requiring hospitalization and surgery. The entire fallopian tube must be removed. Without such surgery, a ruptured fallopian tube usually causes the woman's death. Removal of a fallopian tube cuts in half the woman's chance of becoming pregnant.

If you are a woman who smokes you have more than twice the risk of an ectopic pregnancy as a woman who doesn't smoke. The more a woman smokes, the greater her risk of ectopic pregnancy. One study indicates that women who smoke heavily have a fivefold increase in risk.

Animal studies show that tobacco smoke paralyzes the hairlike cilia that normally sweep a fertilized egg down the fallopian tube and into the uterus. If the fertilized egg cannot reach the uterus, it may implant itself in the fallopian tube. Therefore, some researchers believe that paralyzed cilia in humans may be an important reason for smokers' increased risk of ectopic pregnancy.

In addition, smoking is a risk factor for pelvic inflammatory disease, one cause of ectopic pregnancy. Pelvic inflammatory disease is an inflammation of the fallopian tubes that can interfere with the downward passage of the fertilized egg.

If a woman stops smoking, her risk of ectopic pregnancy will decline. According to one study, after eight years of abstinence her risk will equal that of women who have never smoked.

In Vitro Fertilization

85 A couple undergoing in vitro fertilization reduce their chance of success if either the man or the woman smokes.

A technique called *in vitro fertilization* allows some infertile women to become pregnant. It is used primarily for women with blocked fallopian tubes. The overall success rate of in vitro fertilization is about 21 percent. Couples over 40 years of age have a markedly lower success rate than younger couples.

In vitro fertilization involves giving the woman hormones that stimulate her ovaries to produce multiple eggs. The eggs are then removed from the ovary, combined in a sterile Petri dish with sperm from her partner (or another donor), and incubated. If fertilization of the eggs occurs, several embryos are transferred to the woman's uterus in order to increase the chance of a successful pregnancy.

A couple's chance of success is reduced if either partner smokes while undergoing in vitro fertilization. Studies have demonstrated that, if the woman smokes, more hormones will be required to stimulate her ovaries to produce eggs, and a smaller number of eggs will be harvested. Moreover, some studies have shown that fertilization of the eggs is more likely to fail if either the man or the woman smokes. In one study, the successful delivery of a baby in women undergoing in vitro fertilization was 30 percent in female nonsmokers and four percent in female smokers. Clearly, any couple who plan to undergo the difficult and expensive procedure of in vitro fertilization should avoid smoking.

PREGNANCY AND
BREAST-FEEDING

Hazards to the Unborn Baby

86 **Because a pregnant woman's smoking is hazardous to her unborn baby, if you are a woman who is able to conceive, and are sexually active, you should not smoke.**

If you smoke during pregnancy, you increase your risk of having a miscarriage, a stillbirth, a premature birth, a low-birth-weight baby, or a baby with birth defects. Smoking can also cause your child to have behavior problems and reduced intellectual capacity. These hazards are discussed in detail below.

The health of a fetus developing in the womb depends to a great extent on the health of its mother. If you plan to become pregnant you should eat nutritious food, exercise, get enough sleep, and refrain from using illicit drugs, drinking alcohol, smoking, and exposing yourself to secondhand smoke. If you are able to conceive and are sexually active you should do the same, even if you don't plan to become pregnant. About 50 percent of pregnancies are unplanned.

Smoking is most likely to have a harmful effect on your baby's development early in your pregnancy, when you may not yet be aware that you have conceived. Continuing to smoke, of course, continues to harm your baby throughout your pregnancy. Quitting smoking during pregnancy is far better than not stopping at all, but why take the chance that the developing embryo will already have sustained damage?

Smoking during labor is particularly dangerous for the baby. If a mother stops smoking 48 hours or more before her baby is born, the infant's supply of oxygen will be increased during the critical hours of delivery, improving the baby's chance for a safe birth.

Unfortunately, because tobacco is addictive, only about 30 percent of pregnant smokers stop smoking during pregnancy. This is an extremely important reason for young girls not to begin smoking, or to make every effort to quit before they become sexually active. The lives and health of the most innocent and vulnerable are at stake.

87 Smoking increases the risk of problems with the placenta that can endanger the mother, as well as the unborn baby.

The *placenta* (afterbirth) is a disk-shaped temporary organ that grows inside the uterus during pregnancy. One side of the placenta is attached to the inside wall of the uterus. Out of the other side of the placenta grows the umbilical cord that is attached to the baby. The baby receives nourishment and oxygen through the placenta. After the baby is born, the placenta detaches from the uterine wall and is expelled. Smoking during pregnancy can damage the placenta and result in a low-birth-weight baby who is more likely to die soon after birth.

Smoking also increases the risk of a medical condition called *placental abruption*, in which the placenta partially or completely detaches from the wall of the uterus during pregnancy, rather than after the baby's birth. If there is only a slight detachment, there will be vaginal bleeding and mild discomfort, but the baby will remain healthy. A large detachment is a medical emergency that requires hospitalization.

The symptoms of a large detachment can include heavy vaginal bleeding, severe pain in the abdomen, and shock. The baby may make sudden, violent movements that indicate it is being deprived of oxygen. A large detachment usually results in the baby's death. Blood transfusions may be required to save the mother's life. Kidney failure and blood clots are other possible complications for the mother.

Placental detachment occurs in about one percent of pregnancies and is more common in women over 35, those who have had more than five pregnancies, those who have received a direct blow to the uterus, those with high blood pressure, and those who smoke. A large federal government study concluded that if a pregnant woman smokes a pack of cigarettes a day, she increases her risk of placental detachment by about 40 percent, and that heavy smoking increases the baby's risk of death when placental detachment occurs.

Also more common in pregnant smokers is a condition called *placenta previa*. Placenta previa is the implantation of the placenta over, or close to, the opening at the bottom of the uterus through which the baby will be born. The increasing weight of the uterus and the baby puts pressure on a low-lying placenta, and bleeding may result. The mother may be restricted to bed for the remainder of her pregnancy. Bleeding is sometimes profuse, making blood transfusions necessary. A cesarean delivery is usually performed if the opening is partially blocked. This prevents the early detachment of the placenta during labor that would deprive the baby of oxygen and cause massive bleeding in the mother. A cesarean delivery is always necessary if the placenta completely blocks the opening, because the baby could not be born otherwise.

Placenta previa occurs in about one out of 200 pregnancies. Older women and women who have had several children are more at risk. A pregnant woman who smokes a pack of cigarettes a day is more than twice as likely to experience a placenta previa as a nonsmoker. Some authorities believe that the carbon monoxide in cigarette smoke, which reduces the oxygen available to the baby, may cause the placenta to compensate by growing larger, making it more apt to grow over the opening in the uterus. A woman can reduce her risk of problems with the placenta by not smoking during pregnancy.

88 If you smoke while pregnant, you are twice as likely to miscarry. You also increase the risk that your baby will be stillborn.

Miscarriage, or *spontaneous abortion,* is the delivery of a baby before the twentieth week of pregnancy, when the baby is too undeveloped to live outside the womb. The usual reason for a miscarriage is a defect that prevents the baby's natural development. The defect may be in the genes, but often it is caused by something in the baby's environment in the womb. Pregnant women who smoke expose their unborn babies to carbon monoxide and many other toxic substances. If you smoke while pregnant, you are twice as likely as a nonsmoker to have a miscarriage.

Smoking also increases the risk that a baby who is developed enough to live outside the womb will be stillborn—that is, dead at birth. The more heavily a pregnant woman smokes, the greater her risk of miscarriage or stillbirth.

89 If you smoke during pregnancy you increase your risk of delivering a low-birth-weight baby.

Of all the problems caused by smoking during pregnancy, low birth weight is the most common. In a full-term baby, a low birth weight is a weight below 5.5 pounds. Babies born to mothers who smoke during pregnancy weigh, on average, 5 to 13 ounces less than babies born to mothers who do not smoke. The more you smoke during pregnancy, the lower your baby's birth weight is likely to be. Studies also find lower birth weights in the babies of nonsmokers who are chronically exposed to secondhand smoke.

Nicotine and carbon monoxide are the culprits. Nicotine constricts the blood vessels through which nourishment and oxygen are delivered to the baby in the womb. Carbon monoxide reduces the amount of oxygen in the mother's blood so that less is available to the baby. Low-birth-weight babies are more likely to die. If they live, they are prone to respiratory tract infections and are likely to have slower physical growth and intellectual development. Recent studies indicate that low-birth-weight babies are more likely to be autistic.

The lungs of low-birth-weight babies are especially sensitive to secondhand smoke. In a study of 3,285 babies, the incidence of hospitalization for respiratory disease among babies living in households with smokers was much greater for low-birth-weight babies than for normal-birth-weight babies. Because smokers are more likely to deliver low-birth-weight babies, these unfortunate infants are the ones most likely to be exposed to secondhand smoke after birth.

90 Twice as many premature babies are born to mothers who smoke as to mothers who do not smoke.

A baby born before completion of the 37th week of pregnancy is considered premature. Twice as many premature babies are born to mothers who smoke as to mothers who do not smoke.

A premature baby may not have developed adequately to live outside the womb without special care in a hospital, often for weeks or months. A premature baby is more likely than a full-term baby to suffer birth injury, chronic lung problems, cerebral palsy, mental retardation, infections, jaundice, or anemia. Moreover, about 75 percent of newborn babies who die were born prematurely.

91 Smoking during pregnancy causes some birth defects.

There are many types of birth defects. The cause of about 60 percent of them is unknown. But three common birth defects—cleft lip, cleft palate, and clubfoot—occur more often in the babies of women who smoked during pregnancy than in the babies of nonsmokers. A cleft lip is a fissure in the upper lip, a cleft palate a fissure in the roof of the mouth. Cleft lip and cleft palate sometimes occur together. Clubfoot is a condition in which the baby's foot is twisted out of shape or position. One study indicated that heavy smoking by a pregnant woman increases the risk of clubfoot in her infant about fourfold.

Birth defects of the heart, brain, and intestines are also more common in the babies of smokers. And studies show that smoking during pregnancy may cause the baby to have hearing loss that persists into his or her preadolescent years. Research on the relationship between smoking and birth defects is ongoing.

92 Children of women who smoked during pregnancy are more likely to have behavior problems and reduced intelligence.

Smoking during pregnancy is associated with behavior problems and reduced intelligence in children. Behavior problems include conduct disorder (behavior that is unacceptable in the social environment), hyperactivity, and decreased attention span. Reduced intelligence is reflected in poorer school performance and lower scores on tests of language ability. Moreover, the risk of mental retardation is increased for the children of women who smoke while pregnant.

Studies repeatedly find that exposure to the chemicals in tobacco smoke alters the brain development of unborn animals, so it is no surprise that these same toxins cause behavior and learning problems in human children. And exposure to secondhand smoke during infancy and childhood may increase these harmful effects.

93 If you smoke during pregnancy your fetus will have about the same level of nicotine in his blood that you have in yours. He will spend the first days of his life going through nicotine withdrawal.

Nearly everything in your bloodstream passes through your placenta to your unborn baby. If you smoke during pregnancy, your baby will have about the same level of nicotine in his blood that you have in yours. He will be born addicted to nicotine.

Researchers say that newborn babies of mothers who smoked during pregnancy spend the first days of their lives going through nicotine withdrawal. Nicotine withdrawal is stressful, as anyone who has quit smoking can attest. People withdrawing from nicotine commonly suffer cravings, headaches, anxiety, insomnia, restlessness, and irritability. This is a heavy burden to place on your newborn baby.

Morning Sickness

94 **A pregnant woman with morning sickness can lessen her nausea by not smoking and by avoiding secondhand smoke.**

Morning sickness is the nausea and vomiting that most pregnant women experience, usually during the first half of pregnancy. "Morning sickness" is a misnomer—only rarely are the nausea and vomiting confined to the morning. While morning sickness ordinarily is not serious, it is certainly unpleasant. There is no cure for morning sickness, but a number of things can be done to lessen nausea, including eating small, frequent meals, and avoiding greasy foods, cooking odors, and tobacco smoke.

A woman who has morning sickness should not smoke, and should ask other people not to smoke around her. Not only will this help lessen her nausea, but it will also increase her chance of having a healthy baby.

Breast-Feeding

95 Mothers who smoke are less likely to succeed at breast-feeding.

The benefits of breast-feeding for both baby and mother are enormous. The American Academy of Pediatrics urges mothers to breast-feed their babies for at least a year after birth because:

■ A baby receives antibodies and white blood cells from breast milk that he can't get from any formula. These antibodies and white blood cells boost the baby's immune system and protect him from illness.

■ Breast-fed babies have fewer ear infections, respiratory infections, and allergies than bottle-fed babies.

■ Breast-fed babies are less likely to suffer from diarrhea, bacterial meningitis, or sudden infant death syndrome (SIDS).

■ Children who have been breast-fed have a lower incidence of diabetes, childhood lymphoma (cancer of the lymphatic system), and celiac disease (gluten intolerance resulting in poor food absorption).

■ Breast-feeding may enhance the intellectual development of children.

A baby can develop an allergy to formula, but not to mother's milk. Human milk is the ideal food for babies, providing essential nutrients in the most easily digestible and absorbable form. Unlike formula, the composition and amount of breast milk changes over time to meet the baby's changing digestive capabilities and nutritional requirements.

Breast milk is especially important for a premature baby because his mother produces breast milk that is particularly suited to his needs. A premature baby's immune system is poorly developed, making the baby prone to infections. Breast milk can boost immunity and help prevent infections. The premature baby's gastrointestinal system is also poorly developed, and breast milk is more easily digested than formula and less apt to cause constipation. Constipation can be a serious problem in a premature baby.

Breast-feeding benefits the mother as well. Mothers who breast-feed may reduce their risk of early breast cancer, ovarian cancer, and uterine cancer. In addition, breast-feeding provides a measure of birth control, although doctors advise that a barrier method also be used for more complete protection against pregnancy. But breast-feeding is the primary method of birth control in many parts of the world.

Breast-feeding is emotionally satisfying and helps a mother bond with her newborn. Modern hospitals and obstetrical practices often have lactation consultants who help the mother if any breast-feeding problems arise. Breast-fed babies nurse more frequently than bottle-fed babies, but the mother doesn't have to sterilize bottles or water, or mix and warm formula, often while her baby cries with hunger. The breast-feeding mother need only eat a balanced diet that includes an additional 500 or so calories to compensate for what the baby takes. Formula costs at least twice as much as supplemental food for the mother in an average family budget.

If a new mother smokes, breast-feeding is less apt to be successful. Many studies have shown that smokers are less likely to breast-feed their babies. Smokers who do breast-feed are likely to continue breast-feeding for a shorter period of time. An inadequate amount of breast milk is one reason why smokers stop breast-feeding. In the case of a mother who smokes a pack or more a day, her milk-producing hormone (prolactin) levels drop, causing her to produce less milk. She may have to feed her baby more frequently to stimulate milk production. Smoking also interferes with milk ejection from the breast (the let-down reflex), especially if the mother smokes right before or during nursing. Moreover, a smoker's milk tends to be lower in fat and calories and to have an unpleasant taste, leading in some cases to the baby's dissatisfaction and the abandonment of breast-feeding.

A mother can do nothing more important for her new baby than to give up smoking during the time that she breast-feeds him. The breast milk of a mother who smokes contains nicotine and other tobacco smoke byproducts that can have an adverse effect on the baby. One small study showed that babies of smoking mothers breathed more slowly, had less oxygen in their blood, and had higher blood pressure after nursing than before.

Nevertheless, physicians advise mothers who smoke to breast-feed. A baby who is exposed to toxic secondhand smoke in his home has a special need for the extra immunity afforded by breast milk.

A mother who feels she cannot stop smoking will still help herself and her infant if she cuts back on cigarettes and doesn't smoke around the baby. The fewer cigarettes she smokes, the smaller the chance that breast-feeding difficulties will arise. By smoking as little as possible, and avoiding smoking as long as possible prior to nursing, she will reduce the amount of nicotine, carbon monoxide, and other toxic chemicals in her breast milk. The La Leche League, experts on breast-feeding, say to nursing mothers who smoke:

- Smoke away from the baby, outdoors, or in a separate room.

- Smoke right after nursing sessions.

- Smoke as few cigarettes as possible.

POLLUTION AND SMOKING

Outdoor Air Pollution

96 **Both smoking and outdoor air pollution are bad for your heart and lungs. An episode of high air pollution affects more smokers than nonsmokers.**

Every year, industrial countries generate billions of tons of hazardous materials that pollute the air. Hazardous materials of greatest concern include carbon monoxide, ozone, tiny suspended solid particles, sulfur dioxide, nitrogen oxides, lead, volatile organic compounds, and carbon dioxide. Motor vehicles, industries, and utilities generate most of these hazardous materials. Soil erosion adds dust to the air. Forest fires and volcanic eruptions also add hazardous materials.

Some geographic areas are more subject to air pollution than others, depending not only on local generation of hazardous materials, but also on mountains and valleys, temperature, high and low pressure systems, winds, and sunlight. Air quality may change from day to day, and differs from area to area on any given day. For example, measurements taken on a single September day rated air quality "good" in Baltimore, "moderate" in Los Angeles, and "unhealthy" in Dallas. The government provides daily information on local air quality, ranging from "good" through "moderate," "unhealthy for sensitive groups of people," "unhealthy," "very unhealthy," to "hazardous."

The people most likely to be affected by air pollution are children, the elderly, people who are active outdoors, and people with heart or lung diseases. High levels of carbon monoxide and suspended solid particles are especially bad for people with heart disease. When air pollution levels are rated "unhealthy for sensitive groups of people," or worse, those who suffer from heart disease are advised to limit outdoor exertion and avoid sources of carbon monoxide, such as heavy traffic. Episodes of high air pollution increase the number of hospital admissions and deaths due to heart disease. Smokers are more likely to have heart disease, so an episode of high air pollution affects more smokers than nonsmokers.

While ozone in the upper atmosphere shields life on the earth from the sun's harmful ultraviolet rays, ozone at ground level is a powerful lung irritant that may inflame and damage the lining of the lungs. As with heart disease, an episode of high air pollution increases the number of hospital admissions and deaths among people with emphysema or chronic bronchitis. Most people afflicted with these lung diseases got their illness from smoking. What's more, if you smoke and are chronically exposed to air pollution, particularly ozone, you are more likely to develop emphysema or chronic bronchitis. And air pollution combined with smoking is a probable contributor to lung cancer. So if you live in an area plagued with air pollution, you have yet another reason not to smoke.

Indoor Air Pollution

97 If you live or work in a "sick building" with a high level of indoor air pollution, your health will be doubly jeopardized if you smoke.

Since the 1970s, concerns about heating and cooling costs have led to tightly sealed homes and workplaces. Levels of indoor air pollution have risen accordingly. Indoor air is often far dirtier than the air outdoors. A building with high levels of indoor air pollution is called a "sick building." The occupants of sick buildings may develop a variety of illnesses, including nausea, dizziness, sinus congestion, burning eyes, coughs, rashes, headaches, and respiratory problems.

In homes, formaldehyde fumes are commonly released from carpets, textiles, paneling, or foam insulation, and may contaminate the air. Asbestos fibers may be released into the air from deteriorating insulation on the heating pipes in older homes. Faulty furnaces, cooking appliances, and gas dryers may emit carbon monoxide. Mothballs, incense, candles, and so-called air fresheners and room deodorizers will pollute indoor air. Chlorinated water used in showering or laundering can release chloroform. Humidifiers and dampness can pollute the air with mold or mildew. Aerosol sprays and freshly dry-cleaned clothes can emit pollutants. If the outdoor air is also polluted, materials such as ozone, carbon monoxide, and carbon dioxide may mix with indoor air to increase indoor air pollution.

In office buildings, windows often don't open to admit fresh air, and modern ventilation systems recirculate air to reduce heating and cooling costs. People working in these buildings breathe the same recirculated air again and again.

Without good ventilation and maintenance, carbon dioxide, bacteria, viruses, molds, and irritating dusts can pollute the air.

A parking garage in an office or apartment building can be a source of carbon monoxide unless it is properly vented. As in homes, carpets, textiles, paneling, and foam insulation in office buildings release formaldehyde fumes. Some office machines emit ozone or other fumes. Aerosol containers used to spray furniture polish, paint, window cleaning solutions, disinfectants, and pesticides produce mists that contaminate the air. Some cleaning fluids and industrial strength detergents used in office buildings emit noxious fumes. The Environmental Protection Agency has identified about 1,000 indoor air pollutants.

Of all the potential air pollutants in homes and workplaces, secondhand smoke is probably the most pervasive and dangerous to smokers and nonsmokers alike. Secondhand smoke contains thousands of chemical compounds, plus tiny solid particles. Unfortunately, the federal government has not yet banned smoking in all workplaces, although some state governments have a ban, and a majority of employers ban smoking on their premises or provide separate smoking areas.

Steps can be taken to reduce indoor air pollution and exposure to secondhand smoke. In the home, good ventilation, thorough housecleaning, and proper care of appliances will improve air quality. And, of course, air quality will be much better if nobody smokes inside the house or apartment. At work, employees can band together to insist on measures to improve air quality, including a ban on smoking in the building. If this is unsuccessful, employees can file complaints with the federal Occupational Safety and Health Administration.

If you are a smoker who works or lives in a sick building, your health is doubly jeopardized by breathing toxins with every draw on a cigarette, and by breathing polluted air when you are not smoking. In such a situation, it is vital that you quit smoking.

Radon

98 Exposure to radon in the home adds to the risk of lung cancer from smoking and may multiply that risk.

Radon is a colorless, odorless, tasteless, radioactive gas that is produced in rocks and soil and escapes into the air. Enclosed spaces, such as buildings and underground mines, can trap radon. Radon is known to increase lung cancer rates in underground miners. The air in homes tends to have higher levels of radon than the outside air, although lower than levels in underground mines. The amount of radon escaping into homes varies from one geographic area to another, and even within neighborhoods.

The Environmental Protection Agency (EPA) regards radon above specified levels as a health hazard. The EPA estimates that radon causes about 21,000 lung cancer deaths in nonsmokers every year. If you live in an area known to have high levels of radon, it is vital to have the house tested and take corrective action (sealing the basement, installing vent pipes) if high levels of radon are present. But the U.S. Surgeon General urges all homeowners to have their houses tested for radon. This is especially important if there are smokers in the home.

Smoking plus exposure to radon is a potentially lethal combination. Radon exposure, even at low levels, adds to the already considerable risk of lung cancer from smoking. According to some experts, the risk of lung cancer from smoking is multiplied by the risk from radon exposure.

Occupational Pollution

99 **Smoking may interact with substances you encounter on the job, helping to cause occupational disease, or to make it more severe.**

Many jobs subject workers to dust, smoke, fumes, radiation, or various chemicals that can cause occupational disease. A few examples are coal dust in mining, cotton dust in yarn production, rock dust in quarrying, grain dust in farming, smoke and toxic fumes in firefighting, asbestos in demolition, radon gas in uranium mining, arsenic in pesticide manufacture, and chromium in welding. These substances, and others encountered on the job, can by themselves cause disease. Smoking adds to, or multiplies, the risk from many of these substances.

Exposure to asbestos, radon, arsenic, chromium, nickel, and coke-oven emissions has been linked to lung cancer, especially in smokers. The combination of smoking and inhaling asbestos dust is extremely dangerous. Smokers exposed to asbestos are estimated to be 50 times as likely to get lung cancer as nonsmokers not exposed to asbestos. Fortunately, industries that involve asbestos have improved dust control to reduce workers' exposure. Nevertheless, anyone who has ever been exposed to asbestos should be aware that lung cancer can develop as long as 40 years after asbestos exposure. Not smoking will decrease the risk of lung cancer for people exposed to asbestos.

Radon gas is radioactive and increases the risk of lung cancer in underground miners. Underground mines have higher levels of radon than air at the surface. All ore miners are at risk, but the danger is especially great for uranium miners, who are exposed to high levels of radon. Smoking and exposure to radon act together to increase the risk of lung cancer. Moreover, miners who smoke tend to develop lung cancer at younger ages than those who don't smoke.

Inhaling hazardous substances over time can result in loss of lung function. Silica dust, coal dust, welding fumes, paper dust, wood dust, grain dust, and cotton dust are some of the substances that can cause loss of lung function. For example, *silicosis* is permanent scarring of the lungs caused by inhaling silica (quartz) dust. Road and building construction, mining, stone cutting, quarrying, blasting, tunneling, sandblasting, abrasive manufacture, and pottery manufacture expose workers to silica dust. Early silicosis usually has no symptoms unless the worker smokes. Severe silicosis can be fatal, and not smoking is essential to its treatment.

A coal miner who inhales coal dust over time (usually 15 years or longer) is at risk of *black lung disease*. Symptoms include progressive shortness of breath and a cough that produces sputum. The sputum is sometimes flecked with coal. About three percent of miners who accumulate coal dust in their lungs develop a severe form of black lung disease that may cause death from respiratory failure, heart failure, or infection. Cigarette smoking greatly aggravates black lung disease.

Asthma is a lung disease marked by chronic inflammation of the bronchial tubes and unpredictable acute attacks of breathlessness, wheezing, coughing, and tightness in the chest. Susceptible people may develop asthma as a result of exposure to substances encountered at work (occupational asthma). In the United States, about two percent of people with asthma acquired it as a result of such exposure. More than 200 substances are believed to cause occupational asthma, including grain dust, flour dust, wood dust, paper dust, textile dust, synthetic dyes, latex, gum arabic, pollen, and soldering flux. Smoking appears to increase the risk of developing occupational asthma. A person who has already developed occupational asthma should avoid the substance that triggered it and should not smoke. Cigarette smoke worsens the chronic bronchial inflammation of asthma and is one of the most common triggers of acute asthma attacks.

Chronic bronchitis and emphysema—that is, chronic obstructive pulmonary disease (COPD)—usually occurs in smokers, but may occur in nonsmokers who work in certain industries, including leather, plastics and rubber manufacturing, textile mill products manufacturing, food products manufacturing, agriculture, and construction. Smokers working in these industries are at even greater risk of developing COPD.

OTHER HEALTH HAZARDS OF SMOKING

Tobacco Interaction with Medications

100 Smoking reduces the effectiveness of many medications and is incompatible with others.

The effectiveness of many medications is reduced if the patient smokes. If you smoke and take any of these medications, your doctor will have to monitor you closely, adjusting the dose and watching for complications. Smoking reduces the effectiveness of some bronchodilators used to treat bronchial asthma and chronic bronchitis; anti-arrhythmic medications used to treat heart rhythm disorders; and anticoagulant medications used to prevent blood clots. Smoking can also interfere with the effectiveness of tranquilizers, antidepressants, and insomnia and allergy medications.

Smoking is incompatible with other medications for the following reasons:

- Smoking not only makes high blood pressure worse, it lessens the action of many medications used to treat it, thus requiring a higher dose. High doses of many blood pressure medications may worsen the constriction of the bronchial tubes caused by smoking.

- People with insulin-dependent diabetes, which is fatal if untreated, must regularly inject themselves with insulin. The correct dose is vital. Smoking can decrease insulin absorption and increase insulin requirements by 30 percent. Physicians strongly advise diabetics to stop smoking entirely.

■ Smoking reduces the effectiveness of medications used to treat peptic ulcers (crater-like sores in the wall of the stomach or intestine). Smoking also stimulates the secretion of stomach acid and delays the healing of peptic ulcers.

■ Medications used to relieve angina—that is, heart pain—work by relaxing and dilating arteries and veins so that the heart receives more blood. Nicotine constricts blood vessels, thereby working in direct opposition to angina medications.

■ Smoking may interfere with the actions of medications used to treat *psychosis* (severe mental illness involving a loss of contact with reality).

101 Smoking induces or intensifies the side effects of some medications.

Side effects of medications are those occurring in addition to the desired beneficial effects. Side effects can be harmless, harmful, or even fatal. Earlier sections deal with the side effects caused by smoking in conjunction with hormone replacement therapy, birth control pills, and abortion pills. The following are additional medications with side effects that are induced or intensified by smoking:

■ Digitalis is a medication used to treat congestive heart failure. Smoking can predispose a person taking digitalis to heart rhythm disturbances.

■ Ergot preparations, used to treat migraine and other types of headaches, work by constricting blood vessels, thus restricting blood flow. Chest pain is one possible side effect of ergot; others are numbness, cold, and tingling of the fingers and toes. In extreme cases, gangrene (tissue death) of the fingers, toes, feet, or intestine can occur. The nicotine in tobacco, like ergot, constricts blood vessels and increases the likelihood of side effects from ergot.

■ Certain high blood pressure medications may cause or worsen coronary insufficiency (too little oxygen to the heart) and angina (heart pain). The nicotine in tobacco intensifies these side effects. Doctors recommend that all forms of tobacco be avoided when taking these medications.

■ Regular use of certain analgesics to combat pain and inflammation, such as aspirin and ibuprofen, can cause stomach and intestinal irritation and bleeding. Smokers taking these analgesics are more susceptible to their side effects.

■ Primidone, an anticonvulsant, has a sedative side effect—that is, it can produce drowsiness. Smoking can enhance this sedative side effect and cause a greater level of drowsiness, making activities such as driving or operating machinery unsafe.

■ Pentamidine is a drug used to treat the type of pneumonia that afflicts AIDS patients. Coughing and wheezing are possible side effects of this medication. Smokers are more likely than nonsmokers to experience acute coughing and wheezing when taking pentamidine.

Reduced Exercise Capacity

102 **Regular exercise greatly benefits your overall health. If you smoke, you reduce your exercise capacity.**

Regular exercise benefits your health in many ways. The right kind of exercise improves the function of your heart, lungs, and blood vessels, increases your energy, and prevents bone loss. Exercise increases muscular strength, improves balance, and decreases the risk of falls. Exercise aids in weight control, prevents constipation, and may help lower blood pressure and cholesterol. Exercise appears to boost self-esteem and fight depression. For diabetics, the right exercise helps control blood sugar levels. For people with peripheral vascular disease, it increases circulation to the legs and feet. For people with arthritis, it reduces stiffness.

Studies have shown that smokers are less likely than nonsmokers to engage in regular exercise. One reason is that smokers become fatigued more readily than non-smokers. Your muscles need more oxygen during exercise than they do at rest. Smoking promotes narrowing and clogging of your blood vessels, which results in less oxygen-carrying blood to the muscles. Furthermore, the carbon monoxide in cigarette smoke depletes the oxygen in your blood. Smoking can impair even the exercise capacity of teenagers. High school and college coaches discourage smoking and may not allow students who smoke to be on athletic teams.

A smoker who wishes to begin an exercise program should seek the advice of a doctor, who may order an exercise tolerance test to determine if there is coronary artery disease. If necessary, a special exercise program can be developed. Exercise may help you quit smoking. And smokers who quit find that their capacity for exercise improves, in some cases dramatically.

HIV Infection

103 **Smoking promotes certain diseases in people infected with HIV.**

Acquired immune deficiency syndrome (AIDS) is the end result of infection with the *human immunodeficiency virus* (HIV). The virus destroys the white blood cells necessary for normal immune system function. Tragically, AIDS is now a worldwide epidemic that has been extremely difficult to control, especially in the poor nations of Africa. Risky behaviors such as engaging in unprotected sex and using contaminated needles to inject drugs can result in HIV infection. A person who has been infected with HIV may have no symptoms at first. The time that elapses from initial infection with HIV, to the appearance of symptoms, to progression of the disease to AIDS (diagnosed by the appearance of certain symptoms or diseases) varies greatly from person to person.

A healthy immune system protects the body against infections and cancers. When HIV breaks down the immune system, the patient may become fatigued and feverish, have swollen lymph nodes, lose weight, have night sweats, suffer from chronic diarrhea, get mouth, esophagus, skin, lung, or brain infections, or develop unusual cancers. Recent advances in treatment can delay the progression of HIV infection and prolong survival. But there is no cure for HIV infection.

Like HIV, smoking impairs the immune system, although not to the degree that HIV does. Unfortunately, among Americans infected with HIV, a large number are smokers. Smoking promotes certain diseases in people infected with HIV. For example, HIV-infected smokers who develop lung cancer usually get it at a younger age than smokers without HIV infection—at a median age of 48 years versus 61 years, according to one study. Lung cancers in HIV-infected smokers tend to grow more rapidly and cause death sooner than lung cancers in those without HIV infection.

Smokers with HIV infection are more likely to contract bacterial pneumonia. AIDS dementia, the most common cause of mental decline in HIV-infected people, is more likely in those who smoke. Infection with HIV accelerates the onset of emphysema caused by smoking. A pregnant woman with HIV infection is more likely to pass on HIV to her baby if she smokes.

Thrush, a mouth disease that is common in people infected with HIV, is more likely to occur in smokers. Thrush is caused by a fungus and produces sore, creamy-yellow raised patches on a red, inflamed background. Treatment of thrush is usually more successful in nonsmokers than in smokers. Another mouth disease that often occurs in people infected with HIV, hairy leukoplakia, is also more prevalent in smokers. This disease, caused by a virus, ordinarily appears as a white lesion on the sides of the tongue.

HIV infection and smoking are a bad combination. But if a person infected with HIV quits smoking, his or her health outlook will improve.

Organ Transplants

104 A smoker who needs an organ transplant will be at a serious disadvantage compared to a nonsmoker.

Organs that can be transplanted include the kidneys, heart, lungs, liver, and pancreas. Transplants save thousands of lives each year. The techniques developed over the past few decades have steadily increased the success rate of transplantation, but the supply of organs falls far short of the need. Many thousands of Americans are on organ transplant waiting lists, and many die while waiting. To derive the greatest benefit from donor organs, and to promote fairness, people in need of an organ transplant are carefully screened.

The first step toward receiving an organ transplant is to be put on a transplant center's waiting list. Each center in this country sets its own criteria. Centers evaluate detrimental habits such as smoking or drinking alcohol when determining who gets on the waiting list. A smoker may be rejected outright because smokers' transplants are less likely to be successful. Or a transplant center may require smokers to abstain from smoking for a specified period of time before they can be considered. Some transplant centers periodically obtain random urine samples to monitor candidates' nicotine levels. Close attention may be given to whether smoking caused or worsened the disease that led to organ failure in the first place. In addition, smoking causes illnesses, such as coronary artery disease, that may disqualify a smoker from consideration for a transplant. For example, a person with coronary artery disease would probably be ineligible for a kidney transplant.

Transplanting organs from one person to another is a complex process. The tissue types of the organ donor and the organ recipient must match as closely as possible. Even with a close match, the recipient's immune system must be suppressed with drugs that keep the body from rejecting the transplanted organ. The immune system destroys foreign substances, and it perceives the transplanted organ as a foreign substance.

But immune system suppression may be more dangerous for a smoker. In addition to destroying foreign substances, the immune system destroys cancer cells. A number of studies indicate that, as a result of immune system suppression, the incidence of aggressive lung cancers increases in smokers who have undergone heart transplants.

One study showed that a kidney transplant is more likely to fail if the kidney recipient is a smoker. A pancreas transplantation center says the following to its pancreas recipient candidates:

> **Do not smoke**. Transplant recipient candidates MUST stop smoking. Smoking increases surgical risks and can cause failure of the transplanted organ to function.

Understandably, smoking is of particular concern in the case of lung transplant patients. But transplant centers stress the importance of a healthy lifestyle, including abstinence from smoking, for patients who have undergone any organ transplant.

Cluster Headaches

105 **Many people who suffer from cluster headaches smoke heavily, or did so in the past.**

Cluster headache is a chronic ailment with no known cure. Cluster headaches can be so painful that they have been called "suicide headaches." A cluster headache usually starts suddenly and lasts for an hour or two. Cluster headaches come in groups, or clusters, ranging from two headaches a week to several a day. An episode of cluster headaches usually lasts for six to eight weeks, after which the headaches may cease for several months. Cluster headaches can be severely disruptive to work and personal life.

Many people who suffer from cluster headaches smoke heavily, or did so in the past. Some experts believe that heavy smoking is a cause of cluster headaches. Moreover, if you are prone to cluster headaches, smoking may trigger them.

Urinary Incontinence

106 **If you smoke you are more likely to develop stress urinary incontinence, and a cigarette cough may cause leaking of urine.**

Urinary incontinence is the uncontrollable leaking of urine. There are several types of urinary incontinence, but the most common type is *stress incontinence*. Millions of Americans suffer from stress incontinence, about 85 percent of them women. The pelvic muscles support the urinary bladder and urethra (the tube through which urine drains out of the body). When the pelvic muscles weaken—usually because of obesity, pregnancy, childbirth, pelvic surgery, or low estrogen levels after menopause—stress incontinence can result. Coughing, sneezing, laughing, lifting a heavy object, or exercising can cause a person with stress incontinence to leak urine.

Studies indicate that you are more likely suffer from stress incontinence if you smoke. One study found that women who smoke are more than twice as likely to suffer from stress incontinence as women who have never smoked. Moreover, many smokers develop a constant cigarette cough. Coughing is likely to make a person with stress incontinence leak urine.

Because of embarrassment, some people with stress incontinence withdraw socially. Others try to hide their condition because they know that incontinence is a leading cause of nursing home placement. This is unfortunate because there are a variety of effective treatments, including Kegel exercises, bladder training, and surgery. Hormone replacement therapy (HRT) may be prescribed in some cases. But HRT is not recommended for women who smoke because the combination of smoking and HRT increases the risk of heart attack, stroke, and deep vein thrombosis.

Behavioral Influences

107 Tobacco is a "gateway drug" that often leads teenagers to the use of other drugs, and to other risky behavior.

Tobacco is a "gateway drug" that often leads to the use of other drugs, including alcohol, marijuana, heroin, cocaine, crack, hallucinogens, and inhalants. One large study found that more than 74 percent of teenage smokers drink alcohol, compared to only 23 percent of their nonsmoking peers. The same study discovered that 26.5 percent of teenage smokers use marijuana, compared to only 1.5 percent of teenage nonsmokers. Once teenagers are comfortable smoking tobacco, smoking marijuana becomes much easier for them. Marijuana is the most commonly used illicit drug. Another study found that teenage smokers are 22 times more likely to use cocaine than teenage nonsmokers.

Moreover, teenage smokers are more likely than their peers to engage in other risky behaviors. Studies show that teenage smokers are more likely to engage in physical fights or binge drinking, carry weapons, or have sexual intercourse. One behavioral expert urges parents who discover that their teenager is smoking to be on the lookout for other risky behaviors. And parents who don't smoke can serve as good role models to their children. Children of nonsmoking parents are less likely to smoke.

108 Because of cluster behavior, smokers are also likely to engage in other poor health practices. Conversely, people who quit smoking are likely to develop other good health practices.

A number of studies have concluded that both poor health practices and good health practices tend to cluster. This is called "cluster behavior." Thus, a person who smokes cigarettes is more likely to also engage in other poor health practices, such as heavy drinking. A popular observation is that "smokers drink and drinkers smoke." In the United States, more than 80 percent of alcoholics and drug addicts smoke, compared to 21 percent of the general adult population.

Conversely, people who stop smoking often become committed to a healthier lifestyle and take steps to lower their risk of disease and injury. More than one study has found that people who stop smoking are likely to begin drinking more moderately. Former smokers are also more likely than current smokers to eat properly, exercise regularly, get adequate sleep, undergo regular physical exams, and wear seatbelts. Thus, the tendency toward cluster behavior often enhances the health of people who quit smoking.

ADDICTION AND QUITTING TOBACCO

Nicotine Addiction

109 **Experimenting with cigarettes for a few days or weeks can start a lifelong nicotine addiction.**

Nicotine addiction is a critical public health problem, not only in this country but throughout the world. As shown in the sections above, tobacco takes a tremendous toll on the smoker's health. But in this section there is some heartening information. Although conquering a nicotine addiction is not easy, methods of combating addiction have improved greatly in recent years. You *can* quit. You may have to try a number of methods before you succeed. Most former smokers succeeded on the fifth, sixth, or seventh try. But they did quit, and so can you.

Before you can conquer an addiction to nicotine, you must have a firm commitment to quit. The key to making that commitment is understanding the enormous problems created by smoking and the benefits from quitting that are discussed in this book.

The nicotine in tobacco is addicting, both physically and psychologically. The Surgeon General of the United States, numerous scientific studies, millions of smokers, and common sense tell us this is true. Seventy percent of smokers say they want to quit. They haven't quit because they are addicted to nicotine.

The American Psychiatric Association has a standard definition of addiction that includes the following criteria:

- A great deal of time spent taking the substance (hours each day for the average smoker).

- A persistent desire for the substance (ask any pack-a-day smoker).

- Compulsive use despite known risks (every package of cigarettes sold in the United States contains a health warning).

Researchers have found that smoking alters the chemistry of your brain. This is what causes addiction. Nicotine affects brain chemicals that regulate alertness, energy, appetite, depression, and pain. Perhaps most importantly, nicotine elevates *dopamine,* a brain chemical that causes the sensation of pleasure. In this way nicotine is similar to other addictive substances such as alcohol, cocaine, and heroin.

Over time, the smoker's brain adjusts the level of dopamine downward so that more nicotine is needed to produce the same pleasurable effect. Scientists believe that the brain becomes accustomed to operating with a certain level of nicotine and depends on nicotine to produce normal levels of dopamine and other brain chemicals. Nicotine withdrawal then causes distress. While people may begin smoking for pleasure, those who become addicted smoke primarily to avoid the unpleasant effects of nicotine withdrawal.

Individuals differ in their vulnerability to nicotine addiction. Experimenting with cigarettes for a few days or weeks results in addiction for some people—and there is no way to know how vulnerable you are until you are addicted. Studies show that teens become addicted much more quickly than older people. One study showed that some young people who smoke only a few cigarettes a week have the same symptoms of addiction as adults who smoke a pack a day. And children who begin smoking before age 12 are more likely to become heavy smokers than those who begin later.

Nicotine addiction nearly always starts when people are young. Up to 90 percent of adult American smokers started smoking between the ages of 11 and 18. Every day, thousands of Americans under age 18 try cigarette smoking for the first time and many become daily smokers. Despite laws in all 50 states prohibiting the sale of cigarettes to minors, there are many ways for minors to obtain them. Young people buy cigarettes from vending machines or from older friends. Some steal them from stores or from their parents, or present false proof of age to retailers. And some retailers don't even ask for proof of age because laws forbidding the sale of cigarettes to minors are often poorly enforced.

Beginning smokers start because they think it's a sophisticated thing to do, or because their parents or friends smoke. Tobacco advertising, or seeing actors smoke in movies, convince many that smoking is glamorous, fun, and "cool." Beginning smokers usually know that smoking is "bad for you" but almost all believe that they can stop whenever they want. Unfortunately, becoming addicted is much easier than they think. And most young smokers who become addicted wish that they had never started smoking.

110 If you are addicted to nicotine you may be unable to smoke when a craving strikes.

Anyone who is addicted to nicotine has a nagging fear of being unable to smoke when the craving sets in. The craving for a smoke often begins within half an hour after the last drag on a cigarette. Running out of cigarettes where they are not available is one problem. Being unable to find a place to smoke is another.

Smokers are not allowed to smoke in an increasing number of places. Many employers restrict or ban smoking in the workplace, often in order to avoid nonsmoking employees' complaints (or lawsuits) regarding secondhand smoke. Federal law does not permit smoking in workplaces on United States military bases and on most Naval vessels. Hospitals have "No Smoking" signs.

Smoking is commonly prohibited in airplanes, trains, buses, and subways. Some states, municipalities, or restaurant owners ban smoking in restaurants. Smoking in bars is not permitted in some states. Most states have eliminated or severely limited smoking in prisons and jails. The Texas Board of Criminal Justice has banned smoking in Texas prisons, eliminating even a condemned prisoner's right to a last cigarette before his execution.

By law, public schools and some private schools must prohibit smoking. Smoking is not allowed in most courthouses, retail stores, taxis, childcare centers, theaters, playgrounds, rental cars, museums, libraries, churches, doctors' offices, airports, gymnasiums, hotel lobbies, elevators, and health clubs. More and more colleges are banning smoking on campus. Some hotels ban smoking in all of their rooms. Smoking outdoors within a specified number of feet of a doorway to a public building may be prohibited. Parks and beaches are becoming smoke-free. Some farmer's markets have banned smoking. The majority of people do not allow smoking in their homes. Smoking in automobiles is prohibited in some jurisdictions if children are passengers. Smokers who travel find smoking restrictions in many countries that used to permit smoking everywhere.

Because of smoking restrictions, smokers stand on sidewalks, fire escapes, rooftops, decks, and balconies, desperately puffing on cigarettes in the rain, snow, wind, cold, or heat. Smokers stuck for hours in meetings find that they can't concentrate because of nicotine cravings. Smokers seated in smoke-free stadiums or theaters miss part of the entertainment when they exit for a smoke. Hospitalized smokers dressed in hospital gowns, and hooked to intravenous drip bags, wheel the device holding the intravenous drip bag outdoors so that they can get their nicotine fix.

The rapidly shrinking number of places where smokers can satisfy their nicotine cravings unquestionably makes life more difficult for them. However, smoking restrictions accomplish their important goal of protecting nonsmokers from secondhand smoke. Moreover, smoking restrictions make it easier for many smokers to quit because they are forced to smoke less often—and the less often you smoke, the easier it is to quit. Much of the decline in smoking in the United States—from 43 percent of adults who smoke to a little over 20 percent—has resulted from smoking restrictions.

111 Addiction to nicotine may cause you to lose self-respect.

As with other addictions, nicotine addiction sometimes causes people to act in ways that offend their own sense of morality or dignity. A teenage smoker who wouldn't steal anything else may shoplift cigarettes. A smoker working in a smoke-free workplace might sneak a smoke in a toilet stall when the weather is too bad to smoke outside, or time is too short. An otherwise conscientious college student might cut a class in order to smoke.

Smoking makes many people feel that they are weak-willed. One candid smoker described the loss of dignity she felt as she rummaged through the cigarette butts in her fireplace trying to find one long enough to light up again. Another described her mortification when her grown son caught her sneaking a smoke in his basement after she had promised him that she would quit. And a newspaper report tells of a man who confessed to murder in exchange for cigarettes that the police gave him!

The loss of self-respect that results from nicotine addiction should make anyone who is not already addicted think twice before experimenting with cigarettes. Conversely, a smoker who quits smoking has every right to feel proud of the accomplishment.

112 Nicotine addiction wastes your time—and your employer's time.

If you smoke a pack of cigarettes a day, you likely spend one and one-half to two hours a day smoking. Because employers have increasingly banned smoking indoors to protect nonsmokers from secondhand smoke, you may have to spend much of this smoking time outside—regardless of the weather. Too many smoke breaks can result in disciplinary action, or make your boss perceive you as a poor candidate for promotion. Employers usually see smoking as a waste of the time that they are paying for. For them, smoking translates into reduced productivity.

In many families, husband and wife both work, and time spent together is precious. But if you are conscientious about protecting your spouse and children from secondhand smoke, you satisfy your nicotine addiction by smoking away from them, and spend your smoking time alone.

Do the math. Calculate how much time you spend smoking in a year. Then consider what else you could do with that time if you quit.

Quitting Tobacco

113 **Many smokers try to reduce their risk of tobacco-related diseases by smoking supposedly safer cigarettes, or by smoking less. These methods usually don't work and may actually increase their risk.**

In the 1950s, tobacco companies started manufacturing cigarettes with filters. This was followed by "light" or "mild" cigarettes that are supposed to allow the smoker to take in less tar and nicotine. Recently, they have made cigarettes labeled "natural" or "additive free." Slow-burning cigarettes are another recent addition to the market. By smoking these supposedly safer cigarettes, many smokers hope to be able to keep on smoking with less risk of tobacco-related diseases.

Other smokers think that they can lower their risk by cutting down on the number of cigarettes they smoke, or by switching to cigars, a pipe, or a hookah. These methods usually don't work and some methods may actually increase their risk.

Filters for cigarettes were developed to reduce inhalation of cancer-causing tar. Today, 97 percent of the cigarettes sold in the United States are filtered. While filtered cigarettes are probably better than unfiltered ones, they do not make cigarettes safe. Moreover, the filters themselves may be unsafe. Studies have shown that tiny filter fibers are inhaled and lodge in the lungs of smokers. It is quite possible that these fibers cause respiratory disease. In addition, the smoker inhales or swallows toxin-filled charcoal granules that are put into the filters to absorb poisons from cigarette smoke.

To make matters worse, smokers may unwittingly cover the tiny vent holes in the filter paper with their fingers or mouths. Almost impossible to see, the vent holes are meant to reduce tar, nicotine, and carbon monoxide inhalation. Covering them defeats their purpose. Most smokers either don't know that the vent holes are there or don't realize their purpose.

Most cigarettes sold in this country are labeled "light" or "mild," the implication being that they are somehow safer because they reduce the amount of tar and nicotine that smokers inhale. According to scientific studies, *this is an illusion*. The actual quantity of tar and nicotine that a smoker inhales depends on his or her smoking technique. Anyone addicted to nicotine needs a certain amount of it to satisfy nicotine craving, so smokers of "light" or "mild" cigarettes inhale more often and more deeply, or smoke more cigarettes. Studies show that smokers get about the same amount of nicotine and tar when they smoke "light" or "mild" cigarettes as they do when they smoke so-called "full-flavored" cigarettes that are higher in nicotine and tar. Moreover, if a smoker draws smoke deeper into the lungs in an effort to get more nicotine, this can trigger a type of lung cancer that is especially difficult to find and diagnose.

Smokers may buy cigarettes labeled "natural" or "additive free," believing them to be less harmful. This, too, is wishful thinking. The terms "natural" and "additive free" are meaningless. Tobacco naturally contains over 4,000 chemicals, many of which cause cancer, or are poisonous, or both. Pesticides are applied to tobacco growing in the fields, including tobacco used to make cigarettes sold as "natural" or "additive free."

Some smokers have switched to new slow-burning cigarettes in the belief that they are somehow safer. The National Academy Institute of Medicine formed a committee to study whether any scientific basis exists for claims that such novel tobacco products reduce risk for disease. In 2001, the committee chairman stated, "It has not yet been proved that any of the novel tobacco products on the market today reduce illness or death compared to that caused by conventional tobacco products.... Documenting reduced risk for disease could take a long time since cancer and emphysema, for example, take years to develop."

Some teenagers have begun smoking exotic cigarettes from India or Indonesia, often in the mistaken belief that they are safer than regular cigarettes. The cigarettes from India, called "bidis," come in chocolate, strawberry, licorice, and grape flavors. Bidis are cheaper than regular cigarettes, but they are even more dangerous. Clove cigarettes from

Indonesia, called "kreteks," are no safer than other cigarettes, and deliver more tar.

Some cigarette smokers switch to cigars or a pipe, thinking this will reduce the risk of tobacco-related diseases. Studies reveal, however, that cigars and pipes are just as risky, especially for those who formerly smoked cigarettes. People who have only smoked cigars or a pipe rarely inhale, putting them at lower risk for lung cancer, although they are at high risk for cancers of the mouth and throat. And they inhale secondhand cigar or pipe smoke. Cigarette smokers who switch to cigars or a pipe nearly always inhale the smoke. Because cigar or pipe smoke is even higher in tar than cigarette smoke, switching from cigarettes may actually increase the smoker's risk of lung cancer

Hookah, or water-pipe, smoking has increased rapidly in recent years. Hookah bars can now be found in many places. A hookah is a device used to draw tobacco smoke through water. The tobacco is heated with charcoal. Many people who practice hookah smoking have the mistaken belief that such smoking is safe or non-addictive. They may think that the water filters out all the toxins in the tobacco, but this is not true. The World Health Organization (WHO) has pointed out that water-pipe smoking is not a safe alternative to cigarette smoking. Actually, it is more dangerous. A spokesman for the American Lung Association says that one hour of water-pipe smoking is the equivalent of smoking 100 cigarettes. Hookah smoking can result in addiction to nicotine, even though the water absorbs some of the nicotine. Indeed, the WHO points out that hookah smokers addicted to nicotine may smoke more in order to get their nicotine "fix." Moreover, hookah smokers draw in toxins from the burning charcoal, in addition to toxins from tobacco.

Cigarette smokers hoping to reduce at least some of their health risks often cut down on the number of cigarettes they smoke. But studies show that people who cut down usually just smoke harder to make up the difference in nicotine intake. They wind up inhaling more often and more deeply, and smoking every cigarette down as far as it will burn. When researchers studied a group of heavy smokers who had decreased the number of cigarettes they smoked by half, they found that these smokers had just as many cigarette toxins in their bodies after they cut down as they did before. And most smokers who cut down find that the number of cigarettes starts inching up again. One notable exception is that smoking cessation programs successfully use "cutting down" as one of numerous devices to prepare smokers to quit. In conjunction with keeping a written record of every craving and every cigarette, plus switching brands with every pack to weaken brand loyalty and make smoking "taste bad," cutting down on cigarette consumption can be one tool in an effective arsenal of techniques that help people quit.

Some people switch from smoking cigarettes to using smokeless tobacco (snuff or chewing tobacco) in an effort to reduce risk. Although not as dangerous as smoking, smokeless tobacco use can damage the teeth and gums and carries the risk of mouth and throat cancer. It may also lead to other cancers, heart disease, and stroke. A much better option would be to use nicotine replacement therapy—that is nicotine patches, gum, or other nicotine delivery devices—as part of a smoking cessation program.

114 Quitting is difficult and unpleasant for people addicted to nicotine, an excellent reason not to start smoking.

The tobacco industry has argued that smoking is an activity adults freely choose to engage in. Yet drug addicts and alcoholics who smoke say that it is harder to give up smoking than to give up heroin, cocaine, or alcohol. Smokers seldom succeed the first time they try to quit, but average five to seven serious attempts before they are successful.

While people may begin smoking for nicotine's positive effects on mood, withdrawal symptoms make smoking difficult to quit. Without nicotine, the addicted smoker becomes irritable and anxious. Cigarette cravings may be constant. Memory, concentration, and reaction times may be affected. Smoking cessation may activate depression in people prone to depression.

Physical withdrawal symptoms may include cravings, headache, increased coughing, nausea, sweating, insomnia, irritability, anxiety, restlessness, or hunger. Symptoms vary from one person to the next and may last for weeks, or even months. But being mentally prepared for these symptoms helps smokers succeed in quitting. And gradual withdrawal from nicotine with nicotine replacement products also helps.

Some smokers have difficulty quitting because their social lives revolve around smoking. Many of their friends smoke and may discourage them from quitting. Anyone trying to quit will find it difficult to be around other people who are smoking. Establishing new friendships may be helpful, but quitters with close family members who smoke face an additional challenge.

It is also harder to quit smoking in some locales than in others. For example, in California, smoking is prohibited in almost all workplaces, including restaurants and bars, so a California resident who is quitting won't have to continually smell cigarette smoke or see others smoking. It is no coincidence that California has one of the lowest smoking rates in the nation. By contrast, Nevada, with its 24-hour smoke-filled casinos, has one of the highest rates.

Relapse is always a danger. Contact with people, places, and events associated with smoking can reawaken the craving for a cigarette. Stress is another common trigger for smoking relapse. For example, when one former smoker's house caught fire and he stood watching it burn, someone handed him a lighted cigarette. Although he had not smoked for five years, under the stress of the moment and without thinking he began smoking the cigarette and became hooked again. Former smokers need to anticipate that a stressful situation poses particular dangers and plan coping mechanisms in advance.

Consider addiction to cigarettes a chronic illness that can be managed, but not completely cured. For a former smoker, "having just one cigarette" is never worth the risk. And don't listen to someone who tells you, "I can have an occasional cigarette without getting hooked again—and you can, too." Although a small number of smokers seem able to do this, others will cycle from smoking to nonsmoking and back again most of their lives. A former smoker should treat tobacco the way a recovering alcoholic treats alcohol—avoid it entirely.

The difficulty of quitting is an excellent reason not to begin smoking. Those who never smoke never become nicotine addicts and never have to quit. Although quitting is difficult and unpleasant, remember that it is far easier than suffering from lung cancer, heart disease, emphysema, or other diseases that smoking causes.

115 Despite the difficulty of quitting smoking, millions of people have proved that it can be done.

In the United States, 50 percent of people who have ever smoked regularly have quit. Over 44 million Americans are former smokers. You probably know more than one person who used to smoke and has successfully abstained for years. This book is dedicated to the many former smokers that the author knows.

Quitting isn't easy, but it can be done. It's important to keep in mind that nicotine withdrawal symptoms are temporary. And, unlike withdrawal from some other addictive substances such as alcohol, which can produce life-threatening *delirium tremens* (the "shakes") in chronic alcoholics, nicotine withdrawal is not dangerous. No record exists of a person dying from nicotine withdrawal. But enormous numbers of people die because they continue to smoke.

116 When you decide to quit smoking, there is a great deal of help available.

The most important requirement for successfully banishing tobacco from your life is an absolute commitment to quitting. The primary purpose of this book is to help you build that commitment. Another purpose is to make sure you realize how many resources are available to help you quit.

No single quitting technique works for everybody. Some smokers, especially light smokers, are able to quit "cold turkey." And cold turkey should not be ruled out as a quitting method. But many smokers need some help. Studies show that a doctor's advice to quit smoking is a powerful motivator. So make your doctor your partner. The smokers who have the support of their doctors, or other health care providers, are the most successful in quitting.

In 2008, the United States Public Health Service (USPHS) issued a report urging doctors to aggressively treat a patient's smoking just like any other illness. Doctors are urged to ask all their patients whether they smoke, advise them to quit if they do, and offer treatment to those who say they want to quit. Treatment should include both counseling and medications, as appropriate. The report encourages a culture of health care in which failure to treat smoking constitutes an inappropriate standard of care. Action on Smoking and Health (ASH) has pointed out that a doctor's failure to address his patient's smoking could be the basis for a malpractice lawsuit.

The USPHS urges doctors to consider prescribing combinations of medications that have been proven effective in treating nicotine addiction, unless there is a medical reason not to. These medications include nicotine replacements, including patches (e.g. Nicoderm® CQ®), gum (e.g. Nicorette®), lozenges, inhalers and nasal spray, the antidepressant Zyban (bupropion), and a new medicine called Chantix (varenicline). Nicotine replacements help relieve withdrawal symptoms and cravings. They are designed to be used for a limited period of time by gradually stepping down the dosage. Their use doubles the rate of smoking cessation.

The prescription antidepressant Zyban (bupropion) does not contain nicotine. Rather, it works on brain chemicals to reduce nicotine withdrawal symptoms and cravings. You start taking Zyban one to two weeks before you stop smoking. In a recent study of people attempting to quit, 23 percent of those taking Zyban were smoke-free after one year, compared to 12 percent who did not take the drug. Thus, Zyban has about the same success rate as nicotine replacements.

Experts disagree as to whether smoking causes depression or depression causes people to smoke. However, they do agree that smokers are much more likely than nonsmokers to have a history of depression. Zyban can combat depression if it occurs while you are quitting. Two other prescription antidepressants, clonidine and nortriptyline, may be more effective for some people. An antidepressant can help smokers quit, whether they are depressed or not, but former smokers who are prone to depression may need to continue taking the antidepressant.

A recently developed medication called Chantix (varenicline) reduces both withdrawal symptoms and the pleasurable effects of smoking. Chantix was approved by the federal Food and Drug Administration in 2006. Chantix works in two ways: first, it stimulates the release of low levels of dopamine, and second, it blocks nicotine receptors in the brain. Chantix may make quitting easier, but you will still need motivation and determination. People prone to depression may not be able to take Chantix, as it may cause their depression to become worse.

Adding a comprehensive smoking cessation program to medication will make it more likely that you will be able to quit. These programs teach people who are quitting how to cope with situations that trigger the urge to smoke. In general, the more intense the counseling, the more likely the smoker is to succeed in quitting.

There are many types of smoking cessation programs. Individual therapy, provided by a psychiatrist, psychologist, or other health professional, appears to be the most successful, although group therapy helps many people. Telephone counseling is also effective. Inpatient treatment programs exist for those severely addicted to nicotine. Self-help materials may enable some highly motivated smokers to quit.

Hospitals, churches, employers, schools, and health maintenance organizations may offer smoking cessation programs. The American Cancer Society's Quitline® is a telephone counseling program that can help you in your smoking cessation efforts. The American Lung Association sponsors Freedom From Smoking® cessation clinics and an online program. QuitNet.com offers support in quitting. Support groups such as Nicotine Anonymous help their members stay away from tobacco. You can call 1-800-QUIT NOW or 1-877-44U-QUIT for help from people trained to offer support. Notobacco.org is a website that is especially helpful to teenagers.

Some health insurance plans pay for smoking cessation programs. State legislators should be urged to pass laws requiring all health insurance plans to pay for these programs. In states that don't mandate payment for smoking cessation programs, employers, who provide the majority of health insurance, should be urged to voluntarily include coverage for these programs in their health insurance plans. Such coverage saves the employer more than it costs over the long term because employees who quit smoking have fewer absences due to illness. Also, the employer's insurance premiums will be lower because the cost of treating smoking-related illnesses will be reduced.

A smoker who must pay for his own nicotine replacement medication, antidepressant, or smoking cessation program can include the cost as medical expense for federal income tax purposes. Fortunately, an increasing number of states are covering smoking cessation treatments for Medicaid recipients—a group with a high smoking rate.

When combined with a smoking cessation program, exercise has been shown to help smokers quit. Exercise affects brain chemicals and combats depression. In one study of 300 smokers, half engaged in a vigorous exercise program. They were twice as successful in quitting as those who did not exercise.

The American Cancer Society's Great American Smokeout is held on the third Thursday of each November. Smokeout events take place in businesses and schools throughout the country. Friends urge smokers to stop smoking for just one day. If they get through that day without smoking, they are urged to continue their abstinence until "one day at a time" becomes the rest of their lives. The Great American Smokeout has a surprising rate of success. One study found that 25 percent of those who quit for the entire Smokeout day were still smoke-free one year later.

Experts recommend that people who want to quit smoking try various methods until they find one that works for them. Former smokers swear by many different methods, some of them bizarre:

- One man, who was walking toward an airplane he was about to board, saw a sign on the airport tarmac that said, "No smoking beyond this point!" He took this as a personal command, stubbed out his cigarette, and never smoked again.

- Another man reported that he was able to quit simply by circling a date on the calendar and repeatedly telling himself that he would never smoke again after that date.

- A young woman said that her boyfriend, who wanted her to quit smoking, lit one of her cigarettes, inhaled, slowly exhaled, grabbed her and gave her a long kiss. "He tasted so disgusting, I gave up smoking on the spot," she said.

- One four-pack-a-day smoker was able to quit by having himself locked in a motel room without cigarettes for five days. The motel owners agreed to put a special bolt on the outside of the motel room door.

- Some smokers have booked a cruise on a ship that does not allow smoking.

- One former smoker quit by chewing toothpicks instead of smoking cigarettes.

- One woman whose husband had quit smoking, and was urging her to quit, agreed to go to an isolated mountain cabin with him so that she could wean herself off cigarettes. She says, "After several days I was threatening divorce if he didn't drive me to where I could get cigarettes. Several days after that, I was threatening murder. But at the end of the two weeks we were there, I was thanking him for standing firm, and I haven't smoked since."

Hypnosis or acupuncture seems to work for some smokers. Working in a smoke-free workplace has helped many smokers quit.

Experts counsel people trying to quit smoking to see a relapse as part of the learning process, rather than as a failure. A number of serious attempts to quit may be necessary before you are successful in permanently quitting. One former smoker says, "I looked on these lapses not as a disgrace or proof that I would never succeed, but as a useful experience and a reminder that it was not possible to smoke 'just one cigarette.'"

117 **Fear of weight gain deters some smokers from trying to quit. But you would have to gain 60 to 80 pounds to equal the health risks of continuing to smoke.**

Smoking dulls taste and smell, and decreases appetite. Smoking also slightly increases the rate at which the body burns calories. Many teenage girls and some teenage boys begin smoking to stay slim. The tobacco companies encourage this by linking slenderness and smoking in their advertisements. Cigarettes marketed to girls and women are called "slims," "thins," or "lights." The cigarettes themselves and the packs they come in are long and slim. In cigarette advertisements, the models smoking these cigarettes are slim, lovely, and healthy-looking.

Young people who plan to take up smoking in order to be slim and attractive need to remember that tobacco-stained teeth, bad breath, a smoker's cough, and hair and clothing that smell of stale smoke are decidedly unattractive. Moreover, smoking hampers athletic ability, and athletic ability is an attractive quality in any young person. Studies indicate that most people find smokers less attractive than nonsmokers.

From a health standpoint, smoking to control weight is an exceedingly bad bargain. You would have to gain 60 to 80 pounds to equal the health risks of continuing to smoke one or two packs of cigarettes a day. The average weight gain for quitters is ten pounds.

Moreover, smoking seems to redistribute fat to the abdomen, increasing the risk of atherosclerosis, stroke, high blood pressure, diabetes, and possibly breast cancer. When people quit smoking, fat tends to accumulate on the hips, a safer place to store fat. Unfortunately, fear of weight gain deters some smokers, especially women, from trying to quit.

The ability to taste and smell food improves markedly when a smoker quits, and nicotine withdrawal can increase hunger, especially the craving for sweet foods. Many smoking cessation programs help you devise effective ways to deal with this, so you are prepared with substitutes, like celery and carrot sticks in a portable container, sugarless gum, and inedible items that occupy both your hands and mouth. Experts on smoking cessation advise you not to try to diet at the same time that you are trying to quit smoking. The stress of doing both at once will likely sabotage both efforts. Stop smoking first. You will have a strong sense of accomplishment and renewed physical vitality that will help you vanquish the few extra pounds you might have gained.

Exercise is a good way to keep from gaining weight, and may also help you quit smoking. Exercise, like smoking, increases the rate at which the body burns calories. One study showed that women who participated in an exercise program after they stopped smoking gained half as much weight as those who didn't participate.

The antidepressant Zyban, taken to control nicotine withdrawal symptoms and cravings, may also help prevent weight gain. In one smoking cessation study, people who took Zyban gained three pounds, while those who didn't gained six pounds. Nicotine gum also may limit weight gain, according to some studies.

Many people don't gain weight when they quit smoking, simply because they become more active. A new, healthier lifestyle actually results in weight loss for some former smokers. One study showed that, ten years after quitting, former smokers weigh about the same as people the same age who have never smoked.

Benefits of Quitting

118 **When you quit smoking, you will realize immediate health benefits.**

Twenty minutes after your last cigarette, your blood pressure and pulse rate drop. Eight hours after you quit smoking, the carbon monoxide in your blood drops and the oxygen in your blood increases to normal. Your body will begin to heal itself within 12 hours. Within a few days, your senses of smell and taste may improve noticeably. Your risk of some cancers will begin to decline immediately. Your cigarette cough will disappear after quitting, although it may temporarily get worse as your body rids your breathing passages of debris.

Your heart and lungs promptly begin repairing damage that tobacco smoke has caused. Shortly after quitting, energy usually increases and breathlessness decreases. If you have developed emphysema, your breathing will be easier, and the progress of the disease will be slowed. The immediate benefits of quitting have helped millions of former smokers permanently abstain from tobacco.

119 Every smoke-free day a former smoker's body continues to heal itself. The risk of early death and smoking-related diseases declines as nonsmoking time lengthens.

Shortly after you quit smoking, your risk of early death begins to decline. It continues to decline for 15 years, at which point it may approach the level of people who have never smoked. Your risk of smoking-related diseases also continues to decline as long as you remain a nonsmoker. Your risk of heart disease, cancer, and stroke diminishes. Your risk of death from emphysema lessens. Consider the following:

- Your risk of lung cancer may drop 50 percent after ten years of abstinence from smoking. After 20 years, your risk approaches that of people who have never smoked.

- Your risk of cancers of the mouth, throat, and larynx, as well as cervical and bladder cancer, is reduced after only a few years of abstinence.

- Your risk of heart disease diminishes rapidly within the first year of abstinence from smoking, then declines gradually. After 15 years, it is similar to that of people who have never smoked.

■ Although some studies indicate that it takes 15 years to entirely eliminate your risk of stroke due to smoking, other studies indicate that your risk is eliminated after only five years.

Every smoke-free day, a former smoker's body continues to heal itself.

120 The younger you are when you quit, the greater the health benefits.

Beginning smokers frequently think they are invulnerable, much too young for smoking to do any harm. But smoking begins to damage your body immediately. The longer you smoke, the more damage smoking causes. The younger you are when you quit, the less damage smoking will have caused and the greater your body's ability to repair that damage.

The risk of lung cancer increases the longer you smoke. According to one study, smokers who quit while they are young have only half the risk of lung cancer as those who quit in middle age, and only one-tenth the risk of those who smoke until they are old. Quitting while you are young may also avoid irreversible damage to the lungs from emphysema, to the heart muscle from heart attack, or to the brain from stroke. Those who quit smoking by age thirty avoid the increased risk of early death almost entirely, according to a British study.

Studies show that many teenage and young adult smokers want to quit smoking. Special smoking cessation programs aimed at young people are being developed.

Pediatricians are being urged to help their patients quit. These efforts are vital because studies indicate that younger people have a more difficult time quitting than older people do. Nevertheless, the many young people who have quit smoking prove that it is certainly possible to quit while you are young.

121 Quitting benefits people of any age, including the elderly.

Older smokers frequently assume that the damage has already been done and there is no benefit in quitting. *This is not true.* No matter how old you are, or how long or how much you have smoked, there are genuine benefits from giving up tobacco. Even quitting at age 65 adds two years to a man's life expectancy and almost four years to a woman's, according to one study.

And even a 70-year-old who has smoked for decades will improve his heart and blood vessels when he quits smoking. Eventually, his lungs will return from black to bright pink. His risk of lung cancer will decrease, although it will always be higher than in a person who has never smoked. His rate of bone thinning and osteoporosis will be slowed, and his risk of bone fractures reduced. If he has emphysema the lung damage already done is irreversible, but the progression of the disease will slow down dramatically.

An elderly person who quits smoking will be safer from fire, a danger that is much greater for elderly smokers than for younger ones. As one writer pointed out, "A lighted match or a live cigarette dropped from an old man's shaky fingers can be just as lethal as lung cancer." And elderly smokers are likely to be on medications that make them apt to fall asleep while holding a lighted cigarette.

Elderly people who quit smoking usually find that they have more energy. This can give them more independence and control over their lives. Their medications may be more effective, especially some medications for diabetes, or heart or lung diseases.

In 2000, Medicare administrators, concerned about the billions of dollars that Medicare spends to treat smoking-related illnesses in Americans over age 65, began a demonstration project of smoking cessation therapy aimed at the elderly. The administrators hoped that they could convince the Centers for Medicare and Medicaid Services to make smoking cessation therapy available to all Medicare beneficiaries, but they were only partially successful. Medicare now provides for "eight face-to-face [smoking cessation] visits during a 12-month period if you are diagnosed with a smoking-related illness or are taking medicine that may be affected by tobacco." Drugs to help you quit smoking may be covered by Medicare Part D, the Medicare prescription drug plan. One doctor who works in the Medicare program noted, "The health benefits [of quitting] are substantial, even for people who have smoked for a long time."

Although elderly smokers are less likely to try to quit smoking than younger smokers, when they do try they are more likely to be successful. This is partly because the elderly are more apt to seek help in quitting, an important key to success.

SECONDHAND SMOKE

Exposure to Secondhand Smoke

122 **The separation of smokers and nonsmokers may reduce, but does not eliminate, non-smokers' exposure to secondhand smoke.**

Secondhand smoke consists of *mainstream* smoke that the smoker exhales, and *sidestream* smoke that curls from the end of a burning cigarette. About 85 percent of secondhand smoke is sidestream smoke. The concentration of chemicals that contribute to heart disease and cancer may be 30 times greater in sidestream smoke than in mainstream smoke. Even though this high concentration is diluted into the available airspace around the smoker, the presence of harmful chemicals is significant. What's worse, sidestream smoke contains smaller particles of these chemicals than mainstream smoke. These tinier particles can settle deeper into the lungs and take longer for the lungs to eliminate.

The concentration of secondhand tobacco smoke in an indoor space depends on the size of the space, the number of cigarettes smoked, the efficiency of ventilation systems, and other factors. Tobacco smoke moves rapidly throughout indoor spaces. The separation of smokers and nonsmokers may reduce, but does not eliminate, nonsmokers' exposure to secondhand smoke.

The U.S. Surgeon General and the National Institute of Safety and Health have independently determined that merely separating smokers and nonsmokers in public

184

places, or in the workplace, does not provide adequate protection for nonsmokers. Smoke will spread throughout even a large workplace during an eight-hour workday. In smaller indoor spaces with numerous smokers, such as bars, the concentration of secondhand smoke becomes intense. One study showed that cigarette smoke in bars is many times more harmful than diesel fumes in a city street at rush hour. Bartenders and waiters are especially at risk if they work in a bar or restaurant where smoking is allowed.

But even one person who smokes indoors can significantly pollute the air in a house or apartment. Limiting smoking to one room or opening windows won't eliminate the dangers of secondhand smoke. Air filters, air conditioners, and "smokeless" ashtrays do not filter out the toxins in secondhand smoke.

Far too often, nonsmokers are forced to breathe secondhand smoke in the home, the workplace, the dorm room, or other places. Dr. C. Everett Koop, former United States Surgeon General, likens exposing children to secondhand smoke to child abuse. The 2006 Surgeon General's report on secondhand smoke says, "exposure to secondhand smoke remains an alarming public health hazard." Action on Smoking and Health (ASH), a nonprofit organization that is the legal arm of the nonsmoking community, and its Executive Director, attorney John Banzhaf, III, have worked tirelessly for over 40 years to protect the rights of those who cannot protect themselves from secondhand smoke, but much remains to be done.

And a hazard called "thirdhand smoke" has very recently been brought to the public's attention. Thirdhand smoke is tobacco smoke that settles on hair, clothing, furniture, carpets, drapes, bedding, and other surfaces.

Thirdhand smoke contains many hazardous chemicals that remain in the environment after secondhand smoke has abated. Thirdhand smoke is especially dangerous to people with chronic health problems and to children.

In 2001, the Environmental Protection Agency (EPA) began a campaign asking parents to sign pledges that they will not expose their children to tobacco smoke. Other organizations concerned with the health of children, including the American Academy of Pediatrics and the American Academy of Allergy, Asthma and Immunology, are supporting this campaign. If you want to protect the health of family members, don't smoke inside your home. Guests and people who work in your home should be told that smoking inside is not allowed. An EPA administrator said, "People who smoke inside their homes really have two options: quit or take it outside." But it's best to quit to protect your own health, as well as the health of others.

123 Smokers are likely to be exposed to more secondhand smoke than nonsmokers.

Every time you smoke a cigarette, you are exposed to both the smoke you inhale and your secondhand smoke. Smokers tend to associate with other smokers and thus are also exposed to their friends' secondhand smoke. In some workplaces and public buildings, smokers are restricted to a special smoking room. Even smoking rooms ventilated to the outdoors can become blue with secondhand smoke. Many smokers find this objectionable. They complain about the smell of stale smoke and the lack of fresh air. Fortunately, to avoid smoking rooms, some people quit smoking.

As the public becomes more aware of the dangers of secondhand smoke, more smokers will be required to smoke only in smoking rooms or other segregated places. Although this can be unpleasant for smokers, it is vital to protect the health of people who otherwise would be exposed to secondhand smoke involuntarily.

124 Many people have little or no choice about breathing secondhand smoke.

Avoiding secondhand smoke is sometimes not an option. Children whose parents smoke around them have no way to avoid secondhand smoke. These are the most helpless victims. The 2006 Surgeon General's report states that an estimated 22 percent of children younger than 18 are exposed to secondhand smoke in their homes. And some are exposed to secondhand smoke at day care centers.

Adults also may find it difficult or impossible to avoid secondhand smoke. Waiters, bartenders, and casino workers may be forced to breathe secondhand smoke, or change occupations. Other workplaces also expose employees to secondhand tobacco smoke, but that is changing rapidly. Many state and local laws and a majority of employers prohibit smoking in the workplace. Moreover, many unions support smoking restrictions, or a complete ban on smoking. But until federal law forbids smoking in every workplace, some nonsmokers will continue to be at risk.

A person who is married to a smoker may find it difficult to escape secondhand smoke when the spouse is unwilling to refrain from smoking in the house or car. Even when the spouse always smokes outside, his or her hair and clothing may be filled with secondhand smoke.

Fortunately, bus, train, and airplane travel within the United States is less likely to expose travelers to secondhand smoke than in the past. Foreign travel is another matter. People traveling to foreign countries may find exposure to secondhand smoke unavoidable. Moreover, some foreign airlines and most cruise ships are not smoke-free. But a growing number of foreign countries are combating secondhand smoke.

Some colleges permit smoking on campus and in individual dorm rooms. Nonsmoking college students who live in dormitories that are not smoke-free are exposed to secondhand smoke involuntarily. Also, in some colleges smoking is allowed in the cafeteria and lounges. Taking up residence off-campus, or even changing schools, may be necessary for students determined not to breathe second-hand smoke. Complaints by these students and their parents can help change college policies. Colleges that make all their buildings smoke-free not only protect nonsmokers from secondhand smoke, but also may prevent the ten percent of students who are occasional smokers from becoming addicted to nicotine, and help students who are addicted to nicotine to quit smoking.

Death and Illness Due to Secondhand Smoke

125 **Secondhand smoke exposure is the third leading cause of preventable deaths, exceeded only by active smoking and alcohol abuse.**

Each year, thousands of adults, children, and babies die from causes that can be linked to secondhand smoke exposure. Secondhand smoke exposure is the third leading cause of preventable deaths, exceeded only by active smoking and alcohol abuse. A recent U.S. government report estimated heart disease deaths due to secondhand smoke at 46,000 per year. Lung cancer deaths caused by secondhand smoke total about 3,000 per year.

More babies and young children die each year due to their exposure to parental smoking than to all other unintentional injuries combined. Each year, secondhand smoke kills an estimated 430 babies from sudden infant death syndrome (SIDS). About 2,800 low-birth-weight babies die because their mothers smoked during pregnancy. And an estimated 1,100 babies and young children die from respiratory infections attributable to secondhand smoke exposure.

A smoke-free public environment is possible with the enactment of laws that prohibit smoking in all public buildings, workplaces, schools, and daycare centers. But only you can create a smoke-free environment for your children—by not smoking in your house or car, or by quitting smoking altogether.

126 Nonsmokers exposed to secondhand smoke develop atherosclerosis more rapidly than nonsmokers who aren't exposed.

Atherosclerosis is the buildup of plaque in arteries, narrowing them and reducing blood flow. Atherosclerosis leads to heart attacks, strokes, and peripheral artery disease. Atherosclerosis also can reduce blood flow in arteries supplying the eyes, kidneys, intestines, and other vital organs, resulting in serious illness, or even death.

Most adults have atherosclerosis to some extent, and the severity increases with age. Smoking accelerates the rate of plaque buildup in your arteries. Breathing secondhand smoke also accelerates the rate of plaque buildup in the arteries of nonsmokers. A large study of people aged 45 to 64 found that nonsmokers repeatedly exposed to secondhand smoke have a 20 percent faster rate of plaque buildup. Plaque is made up mostly of cholesterol. One reason that secondhand smoke exposure leads to atherosclerosis is that high-density lipoprotein (HDL), the good cholesterol that helps remove excess cholesterol from your body, is lower in people chronically exposed to secondhand smoke.

Researchers in one study found that nonsmokers between 15 and 30 years old who were exposed to secondhand smoke at least one hour a day for three or more years had artery damage similar to people who smoke a pack of cigarettes a day. The greater the secondhand smoke exposure, the greater the damage. Fortunately, yet another study found that, in healthy young adult nonsmokers, artery damage seems to be partly reversible if the nonsmoker is able to stop his exposure to secondhand smoke.

127 If you are already suffering from heart disease, secondhand smoke exposure can make it worse. If you are a nonsmoker without heart disease, chronic exposure to secondhand smoke increases your risk of developing it by 25 percent.

Heart disease kills more Americans than any other illness. Exposure to secondhand smoke is a risk factor for heart disease. Nonsmokers who spend their workdays in a smoky workplace, or who live with someone who exposes them to secondhand smoke, are most at risk. Secondhand smoke puts your heart at risk because:

- If you are a nonsmoker without heart disease, chronic exposure to secondhand smoke increases your risk of developing heart disease by 25 percent.

- Breathing secondhand smoke is particularly dangerous if you have other risk factors for heart disease, such as diabetes or high blood pressure.

- If you are already suffering from heart disease, exposure to secondhand smoke can make it worse.

- Secondhand smoke increases your risk of blood clots.

Most deaths caused by secondhand smoke are from heart disease. Secondhand smoke also causes nonfatal heart attacks and other heart problems, probably three times as many as fatal heart attacks.

Elimination of secondhand smoke from public places provides an immediate reduction in the number of heart attacks in a population. In 2002, Helena, Montana, passed an ordinance creating smoke-free workplaces, including restaurants, bars, casinos, and bowling alleys. The ordinance was in effect for six months before a legal challenge stopped its enforcement. Doctors in Helena noted a 60 percent reduction in heart attacks during the six months that the ordinance was in force, compared to the previous four years.

Then, in 2003, Pueblo, Colorado, banned smoking in restaurants, offices, and other indoor spaces. In the 18 months that followed the ban, a study showed that there was a 27 percent decrease in heart attacks, compared to the 18 months prior to the ban. Pueblo is a geographically isolated town of 104,000 people, and thus an ideal place for such a study.

After a smoking ban was implemented in Monroe County, Indiana, hospital admissions for heart attacks among nonsmokers were reduced 70 percent! However, there was no drop in such hospital admissions for smokers. There now can be no doubt that smoking bans decrease the number of heart attacks in a population.

128 Nonsmokers who breathe secondhand smoke at home or in their workplace have an increased risk of lung cancer.

The Environmental Protection Agency (EPA) estimates that, in the United States, secondhand smoke causes 3,000 lung cancer deaths in nonsmokers each year. The increased risk of developing lung cancer among nonsmokers exposed to secondhand smoke is about 20 percent. The EPA estimates that each year 800 nonsmokers develop lung cancer from exposure to secondhand smoke in their homes. Nonsmokers employed in smoky workplaces are also at increased risk of lung cancer, the amount of risk depending on the quantity of smoke and the years of exposure. Waiters and bartenders are at particular risk.

A nonsmoker's risk of lung cancer from secondhand smoke is small compared with a smoker's risk. But smokers create their own risk, while nonsmokers involuntarily breathe secondhand smoke. No one should be exposed involuntarily to even a small risk of contracting a disease as deadly as lung cancer.

129 Exposure to secondhand smoke is a significant risk factor for stroke.

Strokes are the third leading cause of death and the leading cause of adult disability in this country. A stroke disrupts the oxygen supply to part of your brain. Strokes are usually the result of a blood clot that blocks an artery supplying blood to the brain, but can also be caused by rupture of a blood vessel that causes bleeding into the brain. Strokes have a wide range of effects, temporary or permanent, minor or severe. These effects may include difficulty in speaking, seeing, or controlling emotions; loss of memory; paralysis; coma; or death.

Recent studies have determined that breathing secondhand smoke is a risk factor for stroke. This is not surprising because exposure to secondhand smoke increases the risk of atherosclerosis and blood clots. One study investigated stroke risk of nonsmokers, and of former smokers who had not smoked for more than ten years. The scientists found that when these people were regularly exposed to secondhand smoke for a year or more, their risk of stroke increased 82 percent. Researchers doing another study found that a nonsmoker's risk of stroke is doubled if his or her spouse smokes. Increased risk of stroke is an important reason to avoid breathing secondhand smoke, and an important reason for smokers not to expose others to their secondhand smoke.

130 Almost all nonsmokers are irritated by secondhand smoke. People who have dry eyes or wear contact lenses are especially sensitive.

Exposure to secondhand smoke can cause eye, nose, and throat irritation, headaches, coughing, wheezing, shortness of breath, hoarseness, or nausea. Many people complain about the unpleasant smell of secondhand smoke. Polls show that most nonsmokers find exposure to secondhand smoke irritating and annoying.

In some studies, eye irritation was the most frequent complaint of people exposed to secondhand smoke. The percentage of people complaining of eye irritation increases as the concentration of smoke and the duration of exposure increases. Anyone who has a lower-than-normal flow of tears, a condition called *dry-eye syndrome*, must be especially careful to avoid secondhand smoke and other eye irritants. People with dry-eye syndrome have irritated eyes with a gritty, burning sensation. Dry-eye syndrome is commonplace, occurring most often in smokers, and in older people, particularly women. As you age, the glands that produce tears also age, the quantity of tears may decrease, and tears may evaporate more quickly. Certain medicines (antihistamines, oral contraceptives, some antidepressants) and some diseases (particularly Sjogren's syndrome, a disease that damages tear glands) also cause dry-eye syndrome.

The eyes of people who wear contact lenses are often especially sensitive to airborne irritants. Contact lens wearers may have to remove their lenses if secondhand smoke irritates their eyes. Unless they have prescription eyeglasses readily available, they have to cope with uncorrected vision until the irritation abates.

Children Exposed to Secondhand Smoke

131 Your baby's risk of sudden infant death syndrome (SIDS) is increased if you smoke during pregnancy, or if your baby breathes secondhand smoke after birth.

Sudden infant death syndrome (SIDS), also called crib death, is the sudden, unexplained death of a seemingly healthy baby younger than one year. In the United States, about 5,500 babies each year die of SIDS. SIDS is the most common cause of death of babies between the ages of 7 days and 12 months.

The death of a baby from SIDS is an unexpected, sudden, horrifying event that leaves parents grief-stricken and often filled with guilt. But parents who have done everything possible to give their baby a healthy start in life may derive some comfort from knowing that they did their best for him. A pregnant woman who gets good prenatal care, and who does not take illegal drugs or smoke during pregnancy, is less likely to give birth to a baby who is vulnerable to SIDS. After the baby is born, the risk of SIDS is reduced if the baby is breast fed, put to sleep on his side or back in a safe sleeping environment, and not exposed to secondhand smoke. Parental smoking appears to be responsible for over one-third of SIDS cases. Smoking is probably the most important preventable cause of SIDS.

132 Babies are more likely to suffer from colic if their parents smoke.

More than ten percent of babies have colic, a disorder marked by episodes of crying, irritability, and what appears to be abdominal pain. Colic usually begins a few weeks after birth and continues until the infant is three or four months old. A baby with colic may have crying spells that last for hours despite the parents' best efforts to comfort her. Colic is not dangerous, but it makes parents feel helpless, upset, and exhausted, decreases their confidence in their ability to nurture their child, and interferes with parent-child bonding.

The few studies conducted on the relationship between parental smoking and colic indicate that babies of parents who smoke are more likely to suffer from colic. A recent study of 3,345 infants found that the prevalence of colic was nearly three times higher among babies of mothers who smoked 15 or more cigarettes a day either during or after pregnancy. The study also found that breast-feeding is slightly protective against colic, although breast-fed babies of smokers are still at higher risk of colic than babies of nonsmokers.

133 Children exposed to secondhand smoke have poorer lung function.

Good lung function is necessary for robust health. People with good lung function tend to live longer than those with poorer lung function. A person with good lung function has elastic lungs with normal lung capacity (the amount of air the lungs can hold) for his or her age, sex, and height, and no narrowing or blockage of the airways. A machine called a spirometer is used to measure lung function. Your lung function is measured by how much air you can inhale and how quickly you can exhale.

Critical stages of lung growth and development occur while a baby is in the womb and during infancy. Exposure to tobacco smoke during these critical stages results in reduced lung function. Exposure when the child is older also causes reduction in lung function, but the reduction is smaller.

Many studies have shown that children and teenagers who have been exposed to tobacco smoke have reduced lung function. The greater the amount of smoke exposure, the greater the reduction in lung function. Thus, one study found that children who smoked and whose parents smoked fared the worst.

134 Babies and children have more respiratory tract infections when they have been exposed to secondhand smoke.

A child's risk of upper respiratory tract infections—that is, colds, sore throats, and laryngitis—is increased when the child is exposed to secondhand smoke. Although these infections are not as serious as lower respiratory tract infections, they can make life miserable for the child and for the parents who takes care of her.

Lower respiratory tract infections—croup, bronchitis, and pneumonia—are also more common in children exposed to secondhand smoke. Numerous studies since the 1970s have reported on the association between parental smoking and lower respiratory tract infections in babies and young children. The risk of these illnesses is 70 percent greater if the child's mother smokes and 30 percent greater if the father smokes and the mother does not.

The Environmental Protection Agency estimates that each year secondhand smoke causes between 150,000 and 300,000 lower respiratory tract infections in children under 18 months of age. These infections make 7,500 to 15,000 hospitalizations necessary and result in the deaths of more than 1,000 babies and children.

If you want to protect your children from respiratory infections, don't smoke around them, and make certain that babysitters, nannies, or day care centers don't expose your children to secondhand smoke. And because smokers have more respiratory infections than nonsmokers—infections that they can pass on to their children—you can improve your own health and protect your children by quitting.

135 Children exposed to secondhand smoke are more likely to get middle ear infections.

The ear has three parts: the outer ear, the middle ear, and the inner ear. The middle ear consists of the eardrum and an air-filled chamber containing a chain of three bones that connect the eardrum to the inner ear. A passage called the eustachian tube leads from the middle ear to the back of the nasal cavity.

Because the eustachian tube connects the nose and middle ear, colds can cause middle ear infections. Children are more likely than adults to get middle ear infections because children's eustachian tubes are smaller. Swollen or infected adenoids are another cause of middle ear infections. Most children will have at least one ear infection by the time they are six years old. In many cases, the middle ear infection recurs, and in some cases it becomes chronic.

A middle ear infection usually causes earache, and may cause temporary hearing loss, nausea, vomiting, diarrhea, or fever. Prompt treatment by a physician can prevent more serious complications, such as permanent hearing loss, mastoiditis (infection of a portion of the bone behind the ear), brain abscess, or meningitis (inflammation of the membrane covering the brain).

A recent U. S. Surgeon General's report states that "The evidence is sufficient to infer a causal relationship between parental smoking and middle ear disease in children." One researcher noted that protecting children from exposure to secondhand smoke is one of the few means of preventing middle ear infections.

136 Exposure to secondhand smoke can cause asthma and make it more severe.

Asthma is the most common chronic disease affecting American children. More than four million Americans under age 15 suffer from asthma, a lung disease marked by chronic inflammation of the bronchial tubes (the air passages in the lungs) and unpredictable, acute attacks of breathlessness, wheezing, coughing, and tightness in the chest that may last from a few minutes to several days. Each year 164,000 children are hospitalized because of acute asthma attacks. Nearly 200 die.

Exposure to secondhand smoke can cause asthma in children, makes asthma more severe, and can trigger acute attacks. Children with asthma must be completely protected from secondhand smoke. The American Academy of Allergy, Asthma, and Immunology encourages parents to sign a pledge not to allow smoking in their homes.

Other Problems Caused by Secondhand Smoke

137 Breathing secondhand smoke reduces your exercise capacity.

Chronic exposure to secondhand smoke can harm your heart and lungs. Secondhand smoke increases the level of carbon monoxide in your blood, reducing your blood's ability to deliver oxygen to your heart and other body tissues. For these reasons, nonsmokers chronically exposed to secondhand smoke have reduced exercise capacity. Even young athletes can be affected. A study of nonsmoking high school athletes found a fourfold increase in the incidence of cough and reduced lung function in those who were exposed to secondhand smoke.

Studies have shown that even short-term exposure to secondhand smoke reduces exercise capabilities in healthy nonsmokers, at least temporarily. One study involved stress testing, which evaluates fitness of the heart and blood vessels. The patient walks on a treadmill or rides a stationary bicycle while the exercise intensity is gradually increased. Healthy nonsmokers underwent stress testing, first in a room with clean air, then in a room filled with secondhand smoke. Time to recovery of the pre-exercise heart rate averaged 8.5 minutes in the room with clean air, but 19 minutes in the room with secondhand smoke. The carbon monoxide exhaled by these nonsmokers was three times as great after exercise in a smoke-filled room, as compared to exercise in a room with clean air. In another stress test study, people reached exhaustion more than two minutes sooner when exposed to secondhand smoke.

138 Chronic exposure to secondhand smoke causes antioxidant depletion, increasing your risk of heart disease and cancer.

Breathing secondhand smoke increases the formation of "free radicals," byproducts created when the body processes oxygen. Free radicals damage cells and cause the body to degenerate over time. Antioxidants in fruits and vegetables help to inactivate free radicals, but these antioxidants are used up in the process. A shortage of antioxidants puts people who are chronically exposed to secondhand smoke at greater risk of heart disease and cancer.

Nonsmokers exposed to secondhand smoke do not have as rapid a depletion of antioxidants as active smokers do. But studies show that they have lower blood levels of antioxidants than nonsmokers who are not exposed to secondhand smoke. One study showed that, on average, blood levels of exposed nonsmokers were 24 percent lower in antioxidants.

If you are a nonsmoker exposed to secondhand smoke, you can replenish your stores of antioxidants by eating several servings of antioxidant-rich fruits and vegetables every day. But an antioxidant-rich diet won't undo all of the harm from secondhand smoke exposure. If you can eliminate the source of secondhand smoke—by changing jobs or roommates, for example—this will be much better for your health.

139 If your pet is exposed to secondhand smoke, its health may be harmed.

Animals, particularly mammals, have body structures similar to humans in many ways. Scientists estimate that the genes of mice and humans are 85 to 90 percent identical. The genes of chimpanzees, our closest relatives, are 98.4 percent identical to the genes of humans. So, just like humans, animals exposed to secondhand smoke can suffer adverse health effects. Household pets exposed to secondhand smoke in their homes are harmed in many of the same ways as family members.

Many household pets spend most or all of their lives indoors. If secondhand smoke is present, they constantly breathe it. Secondhand smoke exposure can cause unhealthy changes in the heart and blood vessels of your pet. It also can cause various cancers and lung diseases.

Cats exposed to secondhand smoke are twice as likely to contract a common feline cancer called malignant lymphoma. One study found that dogs, especially long-nosed dogs such as collies and German shepherds, had a risk of nasal cancer 2.5 times greater when heavily exposed to secondhand smoke. Breeds with short noses, such as bulldogs and Pekinese, are more vulnerable to lung cancer when exposed to secondhand smoke. The same is true of cats with short noses, such as Persians. Dogs and cats with short noses are unable to filter secondhand smoke efficiently before it reaches the lungs.

Birds are especially sensitive to any type of air pollutant. This is why canaries were brought into coal mines before the development of ventilation systems. Canaries are quickly affected by carbon monoxide and methane, gasses that may be encountered in coal mines. As long as the canaries kept singing, the coal miners knew that the air was safe to breathe. Pet canaries and other birds should not be exposed to secondhand tobacco smoke. Secondhand smoke exposure can cause pneumonia or lung cancer in pet birds.

Secondhand smoke can trigger asthma in cats. Feline asthma is more common than most cat owners realize. They often think a cat is trying to expel a hairball when asthma is actually causing the cat to cough, wheeze, and struggle to get its breath. Dogs also can get asthma from secondhand smoke exposure.

And pets don't just *inhale* secondhand smoke. Many pets, especially cats, lick up smoke particles trapped in their fur (called thirdhand smoke) when they groom themselves. The cancer-causing agents in these smoke particles make them more likely to develop mouth cancer. Protecting the health of your pet, who cannot protect itself, is one more reason to quit smoking.

INJURIES

Smoking Material Fires

140 Cigarettes, cigars, pipes, matches, and lighters are the most common ignition sources in fatal house and apartment fires.

Smokers suffer more injuries and injury deaths than nonsmokers. Compared to people who have never smoked, current smokers have a 51 percent greater risk of injury death. The more you smoke, the greater your risk of injury. Injury from fire is an especially great hazard for smokers.

Smoking always involves fire. So smokers and those around them are more likely to be injured by fire, or explosion caused by fire. Fire officials warn that smoking materials ignite hundreds of thousands of fires each year in the United States. A fire requires three things—something that will burn (fuel), air (oxygen), and enough heat to make the fuel ignite and burn (an ignition source). An ignition source is created whenever you light a cigarette, cigar, or pipe. Over the years, smoking materials have provided the ignition source for many millions of fires and explosions.

In the United States, the great majority of deaths from fire occur in houses and apartments. Cigarettes, cigars, pipes, matches, and lighters are the most common ignition sources in fatal home fires. And the victims of a home fire often have nothing to do with starting it. For example, a fire that begins in one apartment may quickly spread to other apartments in the building.

In home fires, small children and the elderly have the highest death rates. Children may not know how to escape a fire. Their impulse may be to hide, rather than to get out of the building. Elderly people may be physically handicapped, confused, unable to hear a smoke detector alarm, or have a reduced ability to smell smoke.

Home fires may begin when a cigarette or match ignites curtains, rugs, or clothing. Or an ashtray left on the arm of an upholstered chair may tip over, igniting the chair. Some fires are started when someone thinks a match is extinguished and tosses it into a wastebasket. Others are ignited when a burning cigarette is forgotten on a nightstand, dresser, or kitchen counter. Still others are ignited by children who are playing with matches or lighters that smokers have left lying around.

Home fires often start when a smoker sitting on upholstered furniture drops a cigarette, igniting the sofa or chair. Or people who smoke in bed may set the bedding or mattress on fire. In many of these cases, the smoker has fallen asleep, or is impaired by alcohol or medication. These types of fires may smolder for several hours, producing deadly gases, including carbon monoxide, that render people unconscious. Smoke inhalation, not burns, kills most people who die in fires.

Working smoke detectors do a good job of alerting people to fire in time to make an escape. But firefighters say that smokers often disable their smoke detectors because the secondhand smoke from cigarettes sets off the alarm.

If laws everywhere required cigarettes to be fire-safe, many home fires could be prevented. Fire-safe cigarettes extinguish themselves two or three minutes after the smoker takes the last puff. By contrast, cigarettes that are not fire-safe continue burning 20 to 45 minutes. It may take only 15 minutes for a smoldering cigarette to set fire to upholstery or bedding. New York was the first state to enact a law requiring that cigarettes sold or manufactured in that state be fire-safe. Some other states have followed suit, but a federal law is sorely needed.

Tobacco companies maintain that they don't want to make fire-safe cigarettes because smokers would be annoyed if their cigarettes went out, and they say that a relit cigarette doesn't taste good. They also say that the furniture and clothing industries should prevent smoking-related fires by manufacturing fire-resistant products. Indeed, these industries have made significant progress in this regard. Nevertheless, many homes still have older furniture that is not fire-resistant. Mattresses manufactured since 1973 are fire-resistant, but older ones are still being used. Moreover, fire-*resistant* does not mean fire*proof*.

If you don't smoke in bed, and don't smoke when your alertness is impaired by alcohol or medication, you are less likely to start a home fire. It is safer yet never to smoke in your house or apartment. But it is also important to be careful when disposing of cigarettes and matches outdoors. A carelessly thrown match or cigarette butt can set shrubbery or a wooden deck on fire.

141 Smoking-related fires in hotels, institutions, and residential facilities cause many deaths and injuries.

Most fatal smoking-related fires occur in houses and apartments, but many such fires occur in other buildings that house people, including hotels, nursing homes, hospitals, board and care facilities, mental institutions, prisons, college dormitories, and barracks. Usually, there are many people in these buildings, so multiple deaths and injuries may occur when they burn.

The number of hotel fires has declined in recent years due to the installation of smoke alarms and sprinkler systems. But fires in older hotels without sprinklers still claim lives. And smoking is the most common cause of fatal hotel fires. Sometimes the tenants of residential hotels die or are left homeless when these structures burn. In 1997, the residential Delta Hotel in San Francisco burned. The tenants—many of whom were elderly and all of whom were poor—were left homeless, some with smoke inhalation injuries. One of the tenants admitted that he was a heavy smoker and that he had apparently dropped a lighted cigarette onto a recliner chair that smoldered for hours before bursting into flame.

Patients in hospitals, nursing homes, mental institutions, and facilities for the retarded typically have physical or mental handicaps that may prevent a rapid escape from a fire. Hospitals in the United States do not allow smoking, but some patients don't follow the rules. In fact, studies indicate that it is common for hospital patients to smoke.

Nursing homes frequently forbid smoking by visitors or staff, but the rule doesn't always extend to residents. In 2003, a nursing home fire in Hartford, Connecticut, started when a resident ignited her bedding with a cigarette lighter. The fire killed 16 residents. Charges were not preferred against the resident who started the fire after it was determined that she was incompetent to stand trial.

Nursing homes are especially vulnerable to fires that start when elderly residents fall asleep holding a cigarette. Many residents are on medications that cause drowsiness. Some have Alzheimer's disease or other types of dementia. Elderly smokers need close supervision, but nursing homes are usually understaffed, making it difficult for workers to keep an eye on residents who smoke. Even with an early warning from a smoke alarm, the nursing home staff may be unable to get immobile or confused residents out of the building in time to prevent deaths and injuries.

Smoking is the third leading cause of college dorm and fraternity house fires, after arson and cooking. In one tragic fraternity house fire, investigators determined that smoking materials ignited something combustible underneath an alcohol bar in the basement. The fire spread and five victims died in bedrooms on the upper floors where they were sleeping. Others were injured when they jumped from the building to escape the fire. Another fraternity house fire started when a couch in the assembly room was ignited with a butane cigarette lighter. This fire killed three students and injured two others.

Buildings that house large numbers of people are required to have fire protection devices such as smoke or heat detectors, fire extinguishers, fire doors, fire escapes, and automatic sprinklers. These have saved many lives. Nevertheless, many buildings, especially older ones, lack such safeguards. The fewer smokers there are in these buildings, the safer the residents are from fire.

142 Smoking materials ignite workplace fires that cause deaths and injuries, destroy businesses, and put people out of work.

Every year in this country, smoking materials ignite thousands of fires that burn stores, offices, industries, and farms. These fires cause deaths and injuries, destroy businesses, and put people out of work. The United States has a long history of workplace fires ignited by smoking materials.

The notorious 1911 Triangle Shirtwaist Factory fire that killed 146 workers, mostly teenaged girls, is believed to have been started by smoking materials. The factory was crowded with workers and with thousands of pounds of highly flammable fabric, rags, and rubbish. Tables and sewing machines were wet with flammable sewing machine oil. The fire marshal concluded that a lighted match started the fire. He said that many cigarette cases were picked up near the fire's origin. This tragic fire led to the creation of new fire and building codes that were adopted throughout the nation.

In 1947, an ammonium nitrate explosion in Texas City, Texas, left 576 people dead and injured 3,500. It damaged 90 percent of the buildings in Texas City. The Federal Bureau of Investigation concluded that a cigarette probably ignited the ammonium nitrate.

In 2007, a furniture store fire in Charleston, South Carolina, killed nine firefighters. The building, which was filled with upholstered furniture, had no sprinkler system. The fire started in an enclosed loading dock. An employee of the furniture store said that the loading dock was used for smoking breaks.

Many businesses and industries involve highly flammable or explosive materials. For example, combustible dusts include plastic dusts, coal dust, wood dust, textile dust, aluminum and magnesium dusts, sugar dust, paper dust, and soap dust. Over 280 dust fires and explosions have occurred during the last 25 years, killing 119 people and injuring over 700. In 2003, an accumulation of combustible polyethylene dust fueled an explosion that destroyed a factory, killed six factory employees, and injured 38. The Occupational Safety and Health Administration has pointed out that the combination of combustible dust, oxygen, and an ignition source, such as lighted cigarettes or matches, are the elements of a tragic dust explosion.

Farms also have highly flammable or explosive materials. Hay, straw, grain dust, poultry feathers, fertilizer, herbicides, and pesticides, as well as gasoline and oil used to run farm machinery, are highly flammable or explosive. Moreover, farms are particularly susceptible to extensive fire damage due to their isolation—far away from fire-fighting equipment, and often with inadequate water to fight a fire. Smoking materials are the leading ignition source for farm fires. Experts on farm safety caution against smoking around flammable or explosive materials, or while refueling farm machinery.

While many employers have smoking rules designed to help prevent fires and explosions, other employers ban smoking entirely. A smoking ban lowers the risk of fire damage to the workplace and lowers the employer's fire insurance premiums. Most importantly, a smoking ban helps protect workers from death or injury caused by a fire or explosion, while also eliminating the health hazards of secondhand smoke.

143 Many clothing fires are ignited by smoking materials.

Smoking materials are a leading cause of clothing fires. Clothing fires tend to cause severe burns. Elderly people and children are most vulnerable to clothing fires.

If a smoker falls asleep holding a cigarette, the cigarette or a hot ash may drop onto clothing, igniting it. Toxic fumes may then make the smoker unconscious. In some circumstances, clothing acts as a wick while the body fat burns like the oil in an oil lamp. Firefighters sometimes find gruesome corpses that have been largely consumed in this manner.

Other clothing fires start when someone has a highly flammable substance (often gasoline, oil, or grease) on his clothing, and then lights a cigarette. These fires can easily be fatal. A workers' compensation case was filed by the widow of a smoker who had spilled gasoline on his trousers, then scratched a match on them to light his cigarette. The case report said he became "a human torch."

Every year, hundreds of children playing with matches or lighters set fire to their own or their playmates' clothing. A child whose clothing catches fire will probably have a strong impulse to run, but running makes the fire burn faster. Children should be taught that if their clothing catches fire they must not run, but instead must "stop, drop, and roll." If parents keep matches and lighters out of the hands of their children, it will prevent many of these terrible clothing fires.

Federal law has governed the flammability of clothing fabric for decades. Nevertheless, clothing fires continue to occur because the law effectively applies only to so-called "torch fabrics" that can be engulfed in flames in seconds. Fabrics of intermediate or normal flammability may still be used to make clothing, although stricter standards apply to children's sleepwear.

For both children and adults, the most danger is posed by loose, 100-percent-cotton clothing that has not been treated to resist fire. Most fabrics will burn, but polyester, nylon, wool, and silk are less likely to ignite than untreated cotton. Using fabric softeners repeatedly will also cause fabric to burn faster. Clothing that is difficult to remove increases the danger of severe burns—for example, clothing that must be pulled off over the head.

You can reduce the risk of clothing fires by wearing clothing that is less likely to ignite, and by eliminating ignition sources. Of course, some ignition sources, such as cooktops, can't be eliminated. But smoking materials can be eliminated from homes and workplaces.

144 Some motor vehicle fires are ignited by smoking materials.

There are two main types of motor vehicle fires—those caused by crashes and those that are not. Each year in the United States, thousands of motor vehicle fires not caused by crashes occur. Smoking materials cause some of these fires.

Fighting a motor vehicle fire is extremely dangerous. Automobiles, trucks, and other motor vehicles are made of numerous synthetic materials that emit harmful or deadly gases when they burn. Vehicle fires generate intense heat. Flames may shoot out ten or more feet. Parts of the vehicle can burst from the heat and shoot lethal shrapnel. Airbags can explode. It is possible, although unusual, for the gas tank to rupture or even explode. Firefighters must wear full protective gear and breathing apparatus when fighting motor vehicle fires.

Motor vehicle fires not caused by crashes usually start in one of three places:

- In the engine compartment, from an oil or fuel leak.

- Under the dashboard, from an electrical short circuit.

- On one of the seats when a smoker drops a cigarette or match, or when a smoker throws a cigarette out the front car window and it is blown back into the car through the rear window.

The best way to prevent smoking materials from starting a fire in your vehicle is not to smoke there. And don't let anyone else smoke there either.

145 Smoking materials ignite many wildland fires, resulting in loss of life and property, as well as environmental damage.

In the United States, forest, prairie, and other wildland fires are on the increase. Global warming—resulting in drought, low snowpack, and early snow melt—has been implicated in this increase in wildland fires. Wildland fires cause deaths and injuries, destroy houses, timber, and animal habitats, and pollute the air.

The many houses that have been built next to wildlands compound the fire problem. These houses may be lost when firefighters are unable to contain a wildland fire. Conversely, a fire sometimes begins in a house and spreads to the wildland. Smoking materials are a common cause of house fires.

Smoking materials are also a common cause of wildland fires. Flammable fuels—trees, brush, dead leaves and branches, grasses, weeds, and tree cones—accumulate naturally. A wildland fire can begin whenever these fuels are dry, and lightning, a campfire, or a cigarette ignites them. Smoking in wildland areas is dangerous, especially in dry weather. For example:

- A cigarette ignited a fire in Yellowstone National Park in 1988 that burned 635 square miles of parkland.

- Fire officials believe a cigarette ignited the 1991 wildland fire in Oakland, California, that caused 26 deaths, 148 injuries, destroyed over 3,000 structures and 2,000 vehicles, and left 10,000 people homeless.

- A 1992 wildland fire in California resulted in property damage of $10.9 million and two firefighter injuries. A carelessly discarded cigarette caused this fire.

- In 1993, a hunter threw away a cigarette that caused a fire in Los Padres National Forest. As many as 3,200 firefighters fought this blaze at one time. Costs of suppressing this fire were an estimated $21 million.

- In 2001, a cigarette tossed from a vehicle caused a wildland fire near San Diego that burned nearly 10,500 acres and destroyed 53 homes and other structures.

We are now in what has been called "the age of mega-fires." Mega-fires are wildland fires that are more frequent than in past years, last much longer, burn much more area, with some that are impossible to contain. The worst wildland fire season in the United States so far occurred in 2006, and the fire season in

2007 was almost as bad. In 2008, drought-stricken California suffered many wildland fires that destroyed homes and other property. Human action—arson, or carelessness with campfires or smoking materials—start most wildland fires.

146 Matches, cigarette lighters, and lighted cigarettes start most of the 100,000 fires that children set each year, often with disastrous results.

Children set an estimated 100,000 fires each year in this country. Fire can get out of control with terrifying and deadly speed. One-third of all children who are killed by fire set the fire themselves. Matches, cigarette lighters, and lighted cigarettes are the ignition sources for the great majority of fires started by children. Children have set clothing on fire—their own, their sibling's, or their playmate's. In their homes, they have ignited bedding, furniture, drapes, and carpets. They have started fires outdoors and in schools. In 2008, a ten-year-old boy accidentally started a wildland fire while playing with matches. This fire destroyed 21 homes and injured at least three people.

Because most have been warned against playing with fire, children are understandably secretive, leading them sometimes to hide in a closet full of flammable materials when playing with matches. Children have set houses afire when they toss a lighted cigarette under a bed or under bedclothes to avoid getting caught smoking. Over half of fires started by children start in a bedroom.

Young children are naturally curious and will almost always play with matches or cigarette lighters if they have the opportunity. A toddler as young as two years old is capable of lighting matches and lighters. Children must be taught never to touch matches or lighters, and to tell an adult immediately if they find them. Some troubled children purposely set fires. Any child with a history of repeatedly setting fires or playing with fire needs professional counseling.

If you don't smoke, your children are much less likely to have access to matches and cigarette lighters. They are also less likely to smoke, and therefore less likely to start fires with lighted cigarettes.

147 Most people have daily contact with flammable or explosive substances that can be ignited by smoking materials.

Homes ordinarily contain many flammable or explosive substances. A match, lighter, or lighted cigarette can ignite these substances, causing a fire or explosion. Some of these everyday "fuels" may not be obvious. Liquor, nail polish, polish remover, rubbing alcohol, petroleum jelly, perfumes, and hair spray are all highly flammable. Women have set fire to their hair when they lit a cigarette after applying hair spray.

Aerosol containers used to dispense many products have labels warning: "Contents under pressure. Do not use or store near heat or open flames." The flammability of most aerosol products is due to the propellants and solvents used to dispense the product, rather than to the product itself. But sometimes the product itself is also flammable or explosive. For example, epoxy paint bears a warning that it contains toluene and xylene, the vapors of which may ignite explosively. Labels that state, "Do not smoke," should be taken seriously. Terrible injuries have occurred when smokers lit up while using these products.

Household cleaners are often flammable. Furniture polishes, metal polishes, wood floor cleaners, concrete degreasers, appliance cleaners and waxes, toilet bowl cleaners, oven cleaners, and fiberglass cleaners may be flammable. Spot removers, dry cleaning fluids, and mothball fumes are hazardous fuels.

Yet more flammable substances are found in basements, workshops, and hobby rooms. Some of these are turpentine, mineral spirits, contact cement, adhesive remover, oil-based paint, varnish, stain, paint thinner, and paint stripper. Some produce invisible, explosive vapors that can ignite at a considerable distance from the container.

Natural gas and propane used in furnaces and other home appliances are extremely explosive and must be treated with caution. A 1999 propane explosion in Iowa killed seven people, injured six others, and completely destroyed a house. If a gas or propane leak occurs, you should extinguish all smoking materials, leave the house, and call the gas company, propane supplier, or fire department.

Outdoor barbeque grills commonly involve the use of charcoal starter fluid or propane cylinders. Smoking while handling starter fluid or a propane cylinder is an obvious hazard. Not so obvious are the hazards of gardening materials, such as flammable weed killers, pesticides, fungicides, and fertilizers. Hydrogen chloride products, used for swimming pool care, are flammable and must be kept away from heat or flame.

Gasoline is commonly used in power lawn mowers, trimmers, garden tillers, snowblowers, and other outdoor equipment. Gasoline vapors are explosive and easily ignited. Invisible gasoline vapors can seek out a spark or flame as far as 50 feet away from the liquid gasoline itself. All smoking materials must be extinguished before refueling any machine powered by gasoline, including, of course, the family car. Every gasoline filling station has signs reading "Warning— No Smoking." In Iraq in 2006, two thieves punched a hole in a gasoline pipeline and were siphoning gasoline, when the gasoline exploded, killing 50 people and wounding 80. One of the thieves had been smoking a cigarette.

Smokers often light cigarettes or smoke without thinking about it. This can be deadly in an environment with many flammable and explosive substances—another reason that it's safer to be a nonsmoker.

148 A person who smokes while using supplemental oxygen risks serious burns.

More than 800,000 Americans receive oxygen therapy— that is, they breathe supplemental oxygen to increase the oxygen levels in their blood. Supplemental oxygen flows from an oxygen source (often a tank) through tubing to a two-pronged device inserted into the person's nostrils, or to a mask, or in some cases into a surgically created opening in the person's windpipe (a *tracheostomy*). Portable oxygen tanks are available for people who are not confined to bed.

Many people with emphysema, chronic bronchitis, lung cancer, or heart failure receive oxygen therapy, usually for most hours of each day and for the rest of their lives. Oxygen therapy improves quality of life. Shortness of breath diminishes. Mental functioning, the ability to exercise, and heart failure may improve. Oxygen therapy prolongs the lives of people with emphysema and chronic bronchitis. The disadvantages of oxygen therapy include expense (although

Medicare and private insurance usually pay 80 percent of the cost for eligible people), inconvenience, and an increased danger of fire.

Oxygen is one of three things that must be present for a fire or explosion to occur, the others being fuel (such as clothing or bedding), and an ignition source (such as a lighted match or cigarette). Oxygen itself is neither flammable nor explosive, although it is necessary to make fire burn. And fire will burn more intensely in an oxygen-rich environment.

The clothing and bedding of a person breathing supplemental oxygen become saturated with oxygen. A minimum distance of 25 feet should be maintained between a person using oxygen and any flame, spark, or other ignition source. Obviously, people using oxygen should not smoke, and no one else should smoke near them. In 2008, in Vallejo, California, investigators concluded that a fire in a senior housing facility was likely ignited when a 68-year-old resident who was using an oxygen tank smoked a cigar. This fire killed three people.

The need for oxygen therapy is usually caused by smoking-related diseases. People receiving long-term oxygen therapy often have smoked for many years, and many of them continue to smoke. Before beginning oxygen therapy, they are told not to smoke around oxygen because of the danger of fire and the risk of serious burns. One burn unit alone averages three such cases a year. Some physicians refuse to prescribe oxygen therapy for patients who will not stop smoking.

149 If fewer people smoke, fewer fires will be caused by smoking materials, and fewer firefighters will be killed or injured.

Firefighting is the most dangerous occupation in the United States. In 2008, 114 firefighters died and tens of thousands were injured while on duty. Firefighters are at risk of heart attack, smoke inhalation, burns, heat exhaustion, electrocution, internal injuries, broken bones, muscle injuries, and post-traumatic stress disorder.

At the scene of a fire, a flashover (the sudden spread of flames over an area) or an explosion may cause firefighter deaths or injuries. Sometimes a firefighter falls or must jump from a building. Or a building may collapse while firefighters are inside. Crashes of firefighting aircraft cause injuries and deaths. Some firefighters are killed when they are overrun by a wildland fire. Firefighting is extremely stressful, strenuous physical work that can result in heart attack, especially if the firefighter is in poor physical condition.

Some firefighter deaths and injuries occur during training exercises or when responding to an alarm. Firefighters must get to fires quickly, often on crowded roads, and some die or are injured in collisions.

Every year, smoking materials ignite thousands upon thousands of fires in the United States. If fewer people smoke, fewer fires will be caused by smoking materials, and fewer firefighters will be killed or injured. If you don't smoke, you decrease the risk to these brave men and women.

And firefighters can decrease their own risk by not smoking. Smoking is a major risk factor for developing heart disease, and it increases stress. The United States Fire

Administration notes: "Stress-induced heart attacks remain the top cause of firefighter deaths. Continued focus on firefighter health and wellness likely may reduce the impact of this killer in the future." What's more, a firefighter who smokes is more likely to suffer lung injury than a nonsmoker because of double exposure to cigarette smoke and to combustion products at the fire scene.

Smoke Inhalation and Burns

150 **Smoking materials ignite fires that cause smoke inhalation injury, the main cause of death from fires.**

In addition to the risk of burns, fire presents another, even greater, danger—smoke inhalation injury. More people die from smoke inhalation injury than from burns. Some people die when they are overcome by smoke and cannot escape the fire. Or there can be a great deal of deadly smoke without actual flames, as when a mattress or upholstered sofa smolders. Fire victims with both smoke inhalation injury and severe burns have a greatly increased death rate, exceeding 50 percent.

Smoke inhalation injures the body in a number of ways:

- Carbon monoxide is a byproduct of combustion, present in every fire. Carbon monoxide in smoke robs body cells of oxygen by taking the place of oxygen in the blood.

- Cyanide gas—produced when plastics, polyurethane, wool, silk, nylon, rubber, or paper products burn— also robs body cells of oxygen. The combination of carbon monoxide and cyanide gas can cause death when either one alone would not.

- Carbon dioxide, a gas that fire gives off, stimulates breathing so that more smoke is inhaled. In high concentrations, carbon dioxide paralyzes the brain's respiratory center, causing death.

- Smoke often contains toxic chemicals. Some toxic chemicals, such as acrolein, cause the formation of free radicals that damage the lining of the throat and lungs. Others, such as ammonia, hydrogen chloride, and sulfur dioxide adhere to the lining of the throat and lungs and form corrosive acids or alkalis. These toxins can destroy the cilia that clear airways, cause the bronchial tubes to go into spasm, or cause the windpipe to swell and close. Injury from toxic chemicals also can result in pneumonia.

- Breathing hot air can burn airway passages. Fortunately, dry air is a poor conductor of heat, so injury from breathing hot air is usually limited to the mouth and throat. But in the rare instances where a person breathes steam, the lungs may also be burned. Steam is an excellent conductor of heat.

Smoking materials ignite many of the fires that cause smoke inhalation injury. Smokers who inhale smoke from a fire fare worse than nonsmokers because they already have carbon monoxide in their blood, and their lungs are already compromised from breathing tobacco smoke. Smokers who have developed emphysema or chronic bronchitis are at especially high risk if they inhale smoke from a fire.

151 Smoking materials are the second leading cause of fires that result in burns.

First-degree burns are limited to the upper layer of skin. They produce redness, tenderness, pain, swelling, and slight fever. Second-degree burns affect deeper skin layers and produce blisters. Third-degree burns involve all skin layers. The surface may be white and soft, or black, charred, and leathery. Deep third-degree burns involve fat, muscle, nerves, and even bone.

The severity of a burn depends on its depth, its extent—that is, the percentage of body surface that is burned—and the age of the victim. Burns are more serious in children under two and adults over 40. The health of the victim, especially the strength of his or her immune system, is vital in surviving a burn.

People who would have died from their burns 20 or 30 years ago often survive now. Highly specialized burn centers sometimes save even the lives of people who have been burned over 95 percent of their body surface. But burns and burn treatments cause a great deal of pain, much of which cannot be relieved with pain medications. Moreover, survivors of massive burns must cope with scarring that disfigures them and limits movement of their joints. Plastic surgery can reduce disfigurement and improve joint movement, although many successive surgeries may be required to achieve this. Usually, physical therapy is also needed to regain as much joint movement as possible. Severe burns take a long time to heal and may require years of treatment. Burn care is among the costliest forms of health care.

Burn survivors suffer emotional pain and often need psychiatric help. Some suffer from post-traumatic stress disorder that results in frightening flashbacks of their ordeal. They may become angry, depressed, and socially withdrawn. In a society that places great value on physical appearance, returning to normal life is difficult for people with disfiguring burns.

Each year, 9,000 Americans are seriously burned due to fires started by cigarettes, matches, and lighters. Smoking materials are the second leading cause of fires that result in burns. Thus, if you smoke, you and your family are at increased risk of becoming burn victims. And, if you smoke, a serious burn is more likely to be fatal.

152 **People can sustain painful burns from direct contact with a burning cigarette, a lighted match, or the flame from a cigarette lighter. If someone is burned by direct contact with your smoking materials, you could be legally liable.**

Direct contact with a burning cigarette, a lighted match, or the flame from a cigarette lighter causes many painful burns. In the United States, more than 5,000 children are burned this way every year. The end of a burning cigarette has a temperature of 900 to 1,400 degrees Fahrenheit. Emergency room doctors see children who walked into a cigarette that was held by a smoker or left burning on a counter. Some of these are burns to the face or to an eye.

Adults also get contact burns. A smoker's careless hand gesture can burn another person standing close by. Both adults and children have been burned when they stepped on smoldering cigarettes with bare feet. If a person is burned by your cigarette, you could be legally liable. And, if you smoke, you are always in danger of contact burns from a hot cigarette ash dropping onto your leg, or a match burning your fingers.

Nicotine Poisoning

153 **Cigarettes, cigarette butts, chewing tobacco, and nicotine patches can poison small children and pets.**

Nicotine is a poison used to kill insects and parasites. Nicotine is more toxic than arsenic or strychnine. And the nicotine in cigarettes, cigarette butts, and chewing tobacco can poison children who eat them. The great majority of children poisoned by nicotine are under six years old. Children six months to two years old are at especially high risk because they tend to put everything they find into their mouths. Chewing tobacco is sweet and may be especially appealing to children.

Eating a single cigarette or three cigarette butts can cause nicotine poisoning in a small child. Symptoms of nicotine poisoning include vomiting, nausea, lethargy, gagging, diarrhea, dizziness, rash, and pale or flushed appearance. High doses of nicotine can cause seizures, low blood pressure, and heart rhythm disturbances.

Any child might find a cigarette butt outdoors. But if you use tobacco and have small children at home, you increase their risk of nicotine poisoning fourfold over homes where cigarettes and other forms of tobacco are not present.

Nicotine patches are also dangerous to children. They are efficient at delivering nicotine through the skin into the blood. To a young child, they may look like adhesive bandages. Children may apply them to their skin or chew on them. Even a used patch could contain as much nicotine as six to eight cigarettes—more than enough to poison a small child. Although most victims of nicotine poisoning survive, if the dose is large enough, it can be fatal.

Dogs and cats occasionally eat cigarettes or chewing tobacco left within their reach. As with children, chewing tobacco is appealing to dogs because of its sweetness. Eating tobacco can be fatal to your dog or cat. Smaller animals are especially at risk.

154 Workers who harvest tobacco can be poisoned by nicotine, an illness called "green tobacco sickness."

Green tobacco sickness is an illness of tobacco harvesters. Nicotine, a poison, is absorbed through the skin of harvesters who come in contact with tobacco leaves that are wet from dew or rain. Green tobacco sickness can cause vomiting, nausea, headache, exhaustion, dizziness, abdominal cramps, breathing difficulty, pallor, diarrhea, dehydration, and fluctuations in blood pressure or heart rate. In extreme cases, the harvesters must be hospitalized. Green tobacco sickness usually lasts from one to three days. The illness often affects more than one harvester at the same time. Some harvesters get sick repeatedly during the harvest season.

Many tobacco harvesters are migrant or seasonal laborers, and some are children. Most cases of green tobacco sickness could be prevented if tobacco harvesters were properly educated about this illness and were provided with chemical-resistant gloves and protective clothing called "rain suits." However, rain suits have their own hazard, namely, heat stress. Working with the tobacco plants only when the plants are dry also protects tobacco harvesters. Although the medical community has recognized green tobacco sickness for decades, many tobacco farmers do little to protect their harvesters. According to a study done in 2000, 41 percent of tobacco harvesters reported having the illness during the harvest season.

In 2009, tobacco companies were pressured into developing training materials to educate tobacco farmers about combating green tobacco sickness. And one large tobacco company said that it will require the tobacco farmers with whom it deals to take measures to reduce their harvester's risk of contracting the ailment. But green tobacco sickness will continue to be an occupational hazard until all tobacco harvesters understand the ailment and its cause, and are given the means to prevent it.

Other Injuries

155 **If you smoke you are at greater risk of falls, the most common cause of injury and a major cause of death.**

Falls are the most common cause of injury and a major cause of death from injury. Falls from heights are especially dangerous, so people who work as roofers, window washers, house painters, or in construction have an increased risk of serious injury from falls. Falls from heights occur at home, too, as when a person tumbles downstairs or off a ladder.

Falls on level surfaces are also dangerous. Many people slip in the bathtub or trip over a throw rug. Falls are the leading cause of injury death in people age 65 and older.

Most traumatic brain injuries in elderly people result from falls. As people age, their veins become increasingly fragile, so that even minor blows to the head may cause bleeding around the brain.

Smokers—even young smokers—are more likely than nonsmokers to fall. There are a number of reasons why this is true:

- Exercise maintains the muscle strength, good balance, and agility that help prevent falls. But smokers are far less likely than nonsmokers to exercise, often because of the heart, blood vessel, and lung diseases that smoking causes.

- Smokers have more strokes than nonsmokers, and people who have suffered a stroke are at high risk of falling.

- Poor vision is a cause of falls. Smokers are more likely to develop cataracts or macular degeneration, conditions that impair vision.

- Insomnia and sleep apnea, more common among smokers, cause drowsiness and inattention that increase the risk of falling.

An elderly person may break a bone simply from falling down on a level surface. Over time, our bones tend to lose density and become more fragile. In a person with osteoporosis, the bones have become so porous and fragile that they fracture easily. Osteoporosis is common in elderly people, and especially in elderly smokers.

Older people most often break bones in the wrist or hip when they fall. A hip fracture—a break in the thighbone just below the hip joint—is especially serious. About 20 percent of people with hip fractures die of complications within a year, 40 percent will need nursing home care, and half will have to use a cane or walker. Studies show that osteoporosis and falls are the major causes of hip fractures. Because smokers are more likely than nonsmokers to have osteoporosis and to fall, they are over 40 percent more likely to break a hip.

156 Drivers who smoke have a 50 to 75 percent greater risk of having a motor vehicle accident.

It is common knowledge that drinking and driving don't mix. But it is also true that smoking and driving don't mix. The reasons are more numerous than you might expect:

- Smoking in a car is a distracting activity that takes the driver's eyes and attention off the road and one hand off the wheel in order to locate, remove, light, smoke, stub out, and dispose of a cigarette. If live embers from a burning cigarette fall into the driver's lap, the resulting distraction and panic can become extreme.

- On the other hand, driving with jitters from nicotine cravings also reduces a driver's concentration—and in some situations, such as heavy rush hour traffic on a freeway, it is not possible to stop for a cigarette.

- Anxiety, stress, and depression are more prevalent among smokers and contribute to driving accidents.

- Smokers have elevated levels of carbon monoxide in their blood. Carbon monoxide in the blood reduces visual acuity, especially at night. High levels of carbon monoxide, according to some studies, contribute to driving judgment errors. If the driver or passengers smoke with the windows closed, the carbon monoxide concentration in the car may become intense, further increasing the risk of a crash.

■ Cigarette smoke in the passenger compartment and smoke residue on the windshield can distort or obscure the driver's vision and increase the glare from oncoming headlights. Irritated, watery eyes caused by tobacco smoke can further interfere with seeing the road clearly.

■ Smokers are more likely than nonsmokers to develop cataracts and macular degeneration—both conditions that decrease vision and increase the likelihood of motor vehicle accidents.

■ Smokers suffer from insomnia and sleep apnea in greater proportion than nonsmokers. Sleep-deprived drivers are dangerous drivers.

■ Because smokers are at higher risk for having heart attacks and strokes, there is an increased chance of either happening while they are behind the wheel— with potentially disastrous outcomes.

Alcohol and tobacco are commonly used together. If you add driving, the combination is likely to be lethal. Smokers are more likely than nonsmokers to drive after drinking. But even sober smokers who drive have a 50 to 75 percent greater risk of being involved in a vehicle crash than sober nonsmokers. And smokers are more likely to be at fault when more than one vehicle is involved in a crash.

There is a drive to pass laws forbidding smoking in cars when children are passengers. While this is a good start, forbidding smoking in all cars would be better. And whenever possible, a nonsmoker should drive.

157 If you smoke, you are about twice as likely as a nonsmoker to be injured at work.

The risk of work injury, and of death from work injury, is higher among smokers than among nonsmokers. In fact, if you smoke, you are about twice as likely as a nonsmoker to be injured at work. And the risk of death from work injury increases along with the increase in the number of cigarettes you smoke.

People with physically demanding jobs, such as construction work, mining, nursing, manufacturing, or military service, are at greatest risk of work injuries. Studies of soldiers in training indicate that smoking is a risk factor for bone fractures, muscle strains, knee and foot injuries, and tendinitis. A large study of workers at manufacturing plants showed that workers who smoked had more than a 50 percent increase in lower back injuries, compared to nonsmokers doing the same jobs. In another study, postal workers who smoked had a 40 percent greater risk of work injuries than their nonsmoking coworkers.

There are several reasons why smokers have more work injuries:

■ Tests show that smokers have less muscle strength and agility, and poorer balance, reflexes, and coordination, than nonsmokers. This makes it harder for smokers to avoid injury.

■ Heart disease, cancer, insomnia, cataracts, and other medical conditions that are more prevalent in smokers affect job performance and increase the risk of injury.

■ Finding a cigarette, lighting it, and disposing of the match, ashes, and cigarette butt are distractions from the task at hand.

■ Smoke-induced eye irritation, blinking, and coughing can cause inattention—and accidents.

■ Nicotine cravings reduce concentration.

■ Smoking materials ignite workplace fires and explosions that injure or kill not only smokers, but also coworkers, bystanders, and firefighters.

158 Smokers are more vulnerable to frostbite than nonsmokers.

Frostbite is injury to your skin and underlying tissues due to freezing. Your danger of frostbite becomes greater as the temperature declines, and the exposure time and wind force increase. If your clothing is improper or inadequate, the danger of frostbite is greater. Extremities and exposed skin are most vulnerable, so feet, hands, nose, and ears are most often affected by frostbite.

Frostbite is dangerously deceptive because the affected body part becomes numb, so that you may be completely unaware of what is happening. The extent of damage from frostbite can range from mild and reversible, to severe frostbite that causes gangrene (death of tissue) and makes amputation necessary. Anyone exposed to temperatures below freezing for an extended time—mountain climbers, skiers, hikers, snowmobilers, hunters, soldiers in combat, lost or stranded motorists, and outdoor workers—can get frostbite.

A person with any form of heart or blood vessel disease is particularly vulnerable to frostbite, and much more likely to suffer severe injury. Therefore, smokers in general are more vulnerable to frostbite than nonsmokers because of their increased incidence of heart and blood vessel diseases.

But even a smoker who does not have heart or blood vessel disease should not smoke before or during exposure to extreme cold. Smoking constricts the blood vessels, hampering circulation and increasing the risk of frostbite. And a person who has frostbite must not smoke. Constricted blood vessels hinder the healing of frostbitten tissues.

PHYSICAL APPEARANCE

Skin, Hair, and Clothing

159 **Smoking spoils your skin, causing premature facial wrinkles, making bags under your eyes worse, and turning your fingers and fingernails yellowish-brown. Smoking also makes you prone to psoriasis, an unsightly skin disease.**

Many young people begin smoking because they see it as glamorous. They may think that smoking will make them appear more attractive and sophisticated to others. Tobacco companies do everything they can to foster these notions. In tobacco advertisements, the Marlboro men and the Virginia Slims women have beautiful skin and radiate health, youth, energy, and glamour. They appear to live adventurous, active lives—skiing, snorkeling, and horseback riding in exotic locations.

The reality is quite the opposite. Smokers age more rapidly and are generally less attractive than nonsmokers. One study found that, on average, long-term smokers look five years older than nonsmokers the same age. Long-term smokers are often described as looking "haggard."

Humor columnist Arthur Hoppe, a former smoker, noted:

Not only do cigarettes kill, but while they're doing so, they smell up your clothes and hair, rasp your throat and redden your eyeballs. From this, we can conclude that they do not, as advertised, lead to romance.

234

And, over time, smoking ages your skin. Your skin is the largest organ of your body. Its job is to keep your body temperature constant and to protect underlying tissues from injury, bacteria, drying out, and ultraviolet light damage. Your skin's thin outer layer, the *epidermis*, is composed mostly of dead skin cells that serve as a protective barrier. Your skin's lower layer, the *dermis*, is composed primarily of a strong, fibrous substance called *collagen*, and of an elastic substance called *elastin*. The dermis also contains blood vessels, nerve fibers, muscle cells, sweat and oil glands, and hair follicles.

Because skin is highly visible, unsightly skin can cause embarrassment and even social withdrawal. Healthy, youthful skin, on the other hand, makes you more attractive to others. In general, smokers have less attractive skin than nonsmokers. Many physicians can identify long-time smokers simply by looking at the skin on their faces. What they term "smoker's face" has prominent lines and wrinkles, gauntness, paleness, grayness, and a mottled look.

Wrinkling of the skin occurs with normal aging as the skin thins and loses elasticity. Smoking speeds up this process, making your skin thinner and less elastic at a younger age. Researchers recently studied the skin of 50 pairs of identical twins. Of each pair, one twin was a lifelong smoker and the other a nonsmoker. The smoking twin had, on average, 25 percent thinner skin than his or her nonsmoking twin.

Smoking decreases blood supply to your skin, inhibiting collagen formation and damaging elastin. Smoking also decreases your levels of vitamin C. Vitamin C is necessary for collagen formation. Moreover, women who smoke have lower levels of the female hormone estrogen than nonsmokers, and low estrogen levels may contribute to aging of the skin in women.

Compounding the problem, smokers often have habitual facial expressions that make wrinkles worse. Smokers tend to squint because cigarette smoke irritates their eyes. Habitual squinting increases "crow's feet" wrinkles at the outer corners of the eyes. One study found that people who smoke heavily are 3.5 times more likely than nonsmokers to have severe crow's feet. Smokers are also likely to get furrows in their upper lips from years of pursing their lips around a cigarette.

Excessive sun exposure is another major cause of wrinkling and, when combined with smoking, the damage is greater than the sum of the damage that each causes. One study found that people who smoke heavily are 4.7 times more likely to be wrinkled than nonsmokers, and people with sun exposure exceeding 50,000 lifetime hours are 3.1 times more likely to be wrinkled than people without excessive sun exposure. The study also found that people who smoke *and* expose their skin to the sun excessively are 12 times as likely to be wrinkled as people who do neither.

Bags under the eyes are caused by normal fat that protrudes, giving a puffy appearance. The skin under the eyes is thinner than skin anywhere else on the body. When this thin skin loses elasticity as a result of smoking, bags under the eyes may become more prominent. Although plastic surgery can help reduce bags under the eyes, this is an uncomfortable and expensive procedure.

Both fingernails and the skin on the fingers of smokers may turn an unattractive yellowish-brown. Discoloration primarily affects the fingers used to hold cigarettes. When a smoker with yellow-brown fingernails quits smoking, the new nails will grow in clear. However, while the nails are growing, part will be yellow-brown and part clear, a condition some physicians call "quitter's nail."

Smoking doubles or triples the risk of getting a common and unsightly skin disease called psoriasis. Smoking may also increase the severity of psoriasis. A person with psoriasis has dry, red patches of skin covered with silvery scales. Psoriasis usually appears on the scalp, elbows, knees, or trunk, but can appear anywhere on the body. Psoriasis can be mild with a few spots of dandruff-like scaling, or severe with large patches. About three million Americans have psoriasis and about 100,000 of them have severe cases. In most people, psoriasis tends to come and go, with no permanent cure, although medications can help the symptoms.

160 Balding is more common in smokers, and facial hair growth is more common in women who smoke.

Thick, healthy scalp hair increases the attractiveness of both men and women. Smokers are more likely than nonsmokers to suffer hair loss. Smoking constricts blood vessels in your scalp, impairing blood supply to the hair follicles. Moreover, toxic substances in cigarette smoke damage the hair follicles. Studies of men who smoke indicate that they are twice as likely as nonsmokers to be bald or balding.

Women who smoke are more likely to have unattractive facial hair. One study found that women who smoke more than a pack a day were 50 percent more likely than nonsmokers to have facial hair. The authors of this study said it is likely that smoking interferes with hormones that govern facial hair growth.

161 If you smoke you are more likely to turn gray prematurely.

Gray hair is widely associated with old age. Most people hope to keep their original hair color for as long as possible, and many are upset when they see the first gray hairs in the mirror. Anyone who wants to avoid premature graying should not smoke. A recent study found that long-term smokers are four times more likely than nonsmokers to turn gray prematurely. The researchers noted premature graying in both men and women smokers, and in all age groups.

Dyeing gray hair is always a possibility, but it is time-consuming, expensive, and must be done repeatedly. Some people, especially men, are embarrassed to have dyed hair. If you don't smoke you are more likely to keep the youthful look of your original hair color for a longer time.

162 A smoker's hair and clothing smell of tobacco smoke, an objectionable odor to most people.

Tobacco smoke permeates hair and clothing, causing an odor that is objectionable to most people. A recent survey of 1,000 Americans found that 90 percent—smokers and non-smokers alike—felt that it was important not to smell of tobacco smoke. More than 43 percent of survey respondents said they would change seats on a bus, train, or at the theater, rather than sit next to a person who smelled of tobacco smoke. And nonsmokers say they resent having *their* hair and clothing permeated with secondhand tobacco smoke.

Many smokers use perfume or cologne in an attempt to mask the smell of tobacco smoke. There are now products on the market advertised to banish the smell of smoke when sprayed on the hair or clothing. But completely eliminating the odor of tobacco smoke is probably impossible for most smokers. The only sure way not to smell of tobacco smoke is to avoid both smoking and exposure to secondhand smoke.

Smile and Breath

163 **If you smoke, you are more likely to have stained teeth, cavities, gum disease, and tooth loss. These can keep you from having a beautiful smile.**

A beautiful smile makes anyone more attractive. White, even, teeth and healthy gums make for a beautiful smile. White teeth promote a youthful appearance because teeth gradually darken as we age. Tobacco smoke also darkens teeth, turning them yellow-brown.

The American Dental Association does not approve of whitening toothpastes used to remove tobacco stains because these toothpastes contain abrasives that may also remove tooth enamel. A dentist can bleach your teeth, but bleaching isn't cheap or always pain-free. And bleaching isn't advisable for people with gum disease, a condition often found in smokers. Moreover, unless you stop smoking, tobacco stains will return.

Studies show that smoking increases the risk of cavities that can lead to tooth loss. When a tooth is lost, other teeth may shift, making the teeth uneven and the smile crooked. Moreover, when a tooth is lost, the underlying bone recedes.

The loss of many teeth leads to a sunken-looking mouth, making the person appear older and less attractive. Smokers are much more likely than nonsmokers to lose their teeth.

Healthy, attractive gums are firm and pink. The gums of people with gum disease are swollen, red, and bleed easily. Diseased gums may shrink away from the teeth, exposing tooth roots. The chemicals in tobacco smoke harm the gums, making smoking a major risk factor for gum disease. Smokers have four times as much gum disease as non-smokers. And smokers' gum disease is more severe and develops at a younger age. Chewing tobacco and snuff also harm the gums.

If you have symptoms of gum disease you should see a dentist, who will provide treatment, plan an aggressive oral hygiene routine, and almost certainly advise you to stop using tobacco in any form. Unless the progress of gum disease is halted through expensive periodontal surgery, pockets of pus may form around the teeth. The bone supporting the teeth may erode, causing teeth to loosen and eventually fall out.

Removable dentures can replace natural teeth and gums. But dentures are not as attractive as healthy, natural teeth and gums. Moreover, removable dentures must be taken out at night in order to rest the gums and keep them healthy. A mouth that has no teeth at night could certainly make a person less attractive to his or her mate.

Dental implants are a newer way to replace missing teeth. A dental implant is a metal device implanted into the jawbone where a tooth is missing. New bone grows around the implant and an artificial tooth is attached to the implant. An implant may replace a single tooth, or several implants can support a bridge or full denture. Dental implants are expensive, but often provide a satisfactory solution to the problem of missing teeth. The most important requirements for a successful implant are a solid jawbone and good gum-healing ability. Smokers are less likely to meet these requirements, so dental implants fail more often in smokers.

If you want to have a beautiful smile, you have five reasons (discolored teeth, tooth decay, gum disease, tooth loss, and failed implants) to avoid tobacco in any form. And if you avoid tobacco, you also avoid spending thousands of dollars in an effort to undo the damage to your smile that tobacco caused.

164 Smokers are likely to have chronic bad breath.

Bad breath, or *halitosis*, is most unappealing. Bad breath can limit your social and professional opportunities. Smoking makes the breath smell of stale smoke, an odor that is offensive, especially to nonsmokers. Smokers are more likely than nonsmokers to have chronic bad breath for several other reasons as well:

■ Smokers are four times more likely than nonsmokers to have gum disease, which is an important cause of bad breath.

■ Tooth decay, also more common in smokers, is another cause of bad breath.

■ Because smokers have more gum disease and tooth decay, they are more likely to lose their teeth and have to wear dentures. Unless dentures are kept scrupulously clean, they trap plaque and food particles, resulting in unpleasant "denture breath."

- Sinus infections (sinusitis) are yet another cause of bad breath. Tobacco smoke irritates the sinus membranes and can result in sinusitis.

For all these reasons, nearly every piece of published advice on avoiding bad breath says, "Don't smoke!" An article in one medical newsletter says, "Tobacco use practically guarantees bad breath." And, as one antismoking slogan points out, "Kissing a smoker is like licking an ashtray."

Other Harm to Smokers' Appearance

165 **Smoking is a major cause of complications and poor results from cosmetic surgery.**

Cosmetic surgery has become more and more popular in the United States. It can correct features the patient considers undesirable, such as a hooked nose, a receding chin, or ears that stick out. As they get older, many people opt for cosmetic surgery that minimizes changes in their appearance caused by aging. Cosmetic surgery can minimize wrinkles, jowls, a double chin, drooping upper eyelids, and bags under the eyes. Procedures such as abdominoplasty (tummy tuck) and breast surgery can give the body more pleasing contours. Men who are going bald may elect to have surgical procedures that remedy baldness, including skin flaps, scalp reduction, and hair transplantation.

Long-term smokers, who ordinarily look older than their nonsmoking peers, may be especially eager to improve their appearance with cosmetic surgery. Unfortunately, smoking is a major cause of cosmetic surgery complications for several reasons:

■ Smoking makes your skin less elastic, and skin elasticity is one factor that makes a person a good candidate for certain cosmetic procedures, including facelift and scalp reduction.

■ Smoking constricts blood vessels in your skin, reducing blood supply to surgical incisions. A reduced blood supply inhibits healing.

■ Smoking reduces oxygen in your blood. Oxygen-poor blood inhibits healing. Thus, healing time is longer and scarring much more noticeable after cosmetic procedures.

Some cosmetic surgery is done with the patient under general anesthesia. Smokers have an increased risk of complications from general anesthesia, including breathing problems, chest infections, and blood clots.

Cosmetic surgeons commonly ask their patients to stop smoking for a specified period of time before undergoing surgery, usually several weeks. Smokers are also cautioned not to resume smoking until a week or two after surgery. Some cosmetic surgeons refuse to do a facelift on a patient who is still smoking at the time that surgery is scheduled. A facelift itself temporarily reduces blood supply to facial skin, and smoking compounds the problem. A patient who does not stop smoking is more likely to have skin next to the incision die and slough off. This is also the case with skin flap surgery, a treatment for baldness in which a section of bald scalp is cut out and a section of hair-bearing skin sewn into its place. Smokers are more likely than nonsmokers to have skin or hair follicles die at the edge of the flap.

If you are considering cosmetic surgery, make the smart move and give up smoking altogether. You will have to forego smoking for several weeks anyway. During that time, nicotine withdrawal symptoms will subside, making continued abstinence easier. Furthermore, in the case of a facelift, the smoother skin that results from the procedure will last longer if you don't resume smoking.

166 Smoking is a risk factor for osteoporosis, which often leads to a hunched posture and, eventually, a disfiguring "dowager's hump."

A straight back and upright posture are attractive qualities in men and women of any age. Osteoporosis thins the bones of the spine. As these bones become more fragile and porous, some people develop a hunched posture that becomes progressively more pronounced, eventually resulting in a disfiguring "dowager's hump." More women than men develop osteoporosis, but many men are also affected.

Smoking is an important risk factor for osteoporosis. Other risk factors include aging, being white or Asian, having small bones, having a low calcium and vitamin D intake, and being sedentary. The more risk factors a person has, the greater the likelihood of developing a hunched posture. Of course, you cannot control your age, your race, or the size of your bones, but you can eliminate some major risk factors if you get plenty of calcium, vitamin D, and exercise—and don't smoke.

167 Tobacco users have the highest risk of disfiguring cancer surgeries.

The beautiful and appealing models in tobacco ads attract many young people to smoking and other forms of tobacco use. How ironic, then, that tobacco users have the highest risk of disfiguring cancer surgeries.

In the United States, 90 percent of mouth and throat cancers are diagnosed in people who smoke or use other forms of tobacco. Nasal cancer is at least twice as common in smokers as in nonsmokers. Surgery to remove tumors in the mouth, throat, or nose may require removal of all or parts of the jaw, tongue, teeth, nose, or lymph nodes along the neck, resulting in emotionally traumatic disfigurement. A person with cancer of the larynx (voice box) may lose the larynx and have a surgical hole cut into the front of the throat in order to breathe.

A few courageous people who have had disfiguring cancer surgeries have become spokespersons against tobacco use. One young baseball player, who had used snuff, lost part of his face because of mouth cancer. He now counsels other ballplayers against tobacco use. A woman who was formerly a beautiful model began smoking to look more convincing in tobacco ads. She lectures against smoking to high school students, despite having lost her larynx to cancer. In a magazine article, she says the "robotic rasp" of her artificial speech commands the students' attention.

Another woman who lost her larynx to cancer has appeared on television, smoking a cigarette through the hole that surgeons cut in her throat. She hasn't quit smoking despite her cancer and the physical disfigurement caused by smoking. Her message gets through to young people loud and clear: *Don't start using tobacco. It has a powerful ability to addict.*

RELATIONSHIPS WITH OTHERS

Public Hostility Toward Smokers

168 **If you smoke, public hostility can make you feel like an outcast and decrease your self-esteem.**

Public attitudes toward smokers are sometimes hostile, and can make you feel like an outcast if you smoke. A large majority of American adults—about 79 percent—don't smoke. As scientific evidence on the dangers of secondhand smoke has accumulated, nonsmokers have become increasingly intolerant of smoking. Nonsmokers complain about their hair and clothing smelling of secondhand smoke. Many are angry about having to shoulder the increased health care costs that result from smoking. Lawsuits are being filed against people who subject others to secondhand smoke. One magazine article noted that, "Where there's smoke, there's ire."

Smokers report that some nonsmokers verbally abuse or even physically assault them. One smoker says a five-year-old accosted him and hissed, "This is bad for you. You're gonna' die." A few smokers in New York City have had the tips of their cigarettes or cigars snipped off by a woman who carries shears for that purpose. Nonsmokers glare at smokers and fan themselves to indicate their displeasure over drifting tobacco smoke. Passersby cast scornful looks at smokers huddled in front of office buildings getting their "fix" of nicotine.

There is a steady stream of negative comments about smokers and smoking in newspapers and magazines:

■ News articles point out that many celebrities, whose smoking in years gone by was considered glamorous and sophisticated, are dead from smoking-related diseases. The list includes Humphrey Bogart, John Wayne, Bette Davis, Sammy Davis, Jr., Steve McQueen, Yul Brynner, Nat King Cole, Lucille Ball, Betty Grable, Gary Cooper, Harry James, Edward R. Morrow, and, ironically, two male models who portrayed the "Marlboro Man" in cigarette ads. In 2009, Alan Landers, who appeared in Winston cigarette ads, and called himself the "Winston Man," died of throat cancer. He also had lung cancer, heart disease and emphysema.

■ A reader complained to advice columnist "Dear Abby" that smokers are "selfish and inconsiderate." Abby replied, "I have little patience and even less compassion for smokers."

■ Smoking is more common among less educated and poorer people. News reports emphasize that much of society now perceives smoking as a lower class habit.

■ Columnist Russell Baker wrote, "Of all the nasty punishments for smoking nowadays, the worst must be the smoker's sense of being a Typhoid Mary."

■ Even a cigarette manufacturer admitted in a magazine advertisement that "The welcome mat is seldom out for smokers."

Public opinion continues to turn against smoking. As one example, in 1982, the U.S. Postal Service issued a stamp picturing Franklin Delano Roosevelt clenching his famous signature cigarette holder between his teeth, but now the Postal Service deletes cigarettes and cigars from the pictures of famous people that it puts on stamps.

In response to public hostility toward smokers, some "smokers' rights" groups have formed around the country. Compared to other rights activists who usually organize massive rallies, marshal public opinion to their cause, and stop government bodies from enacting legislation that abridges their freedoms, smokers' rights groups have been notably ineffective.

Public hostility can decrease a smoker's self-esteem and may be a factor in the high rate of depression among smokers. Quitting tobacco, on the other hand, enhances self-esteem. A former smoker has a right to feel proud of conquering a powerful addiction.

169 Many religions forbid adherents to use tobacco, and may sanction, shun, or expel those who do.

Since ancient times, most of the world's major religions have encouraged followers to take care of their bodies. In Judaism, care of the body is a religious obligation. The Talmud—a collection of ancient rabbinical writings that are the basis of religious authority in Orthodox Judaism—contains all manner of instructions aimed at preventing illness or regaining health. The Christian Bible and Islamic Qur'an likewise have commandments regarding physical health. The Christian New Testament says: "What? Know ye not that your body is the temple of the Holy Ghost which is in you, which ye have of God, and ye are not your own."

Muslims are commanded "...make not your own hands contribute to your destruction..."

Of course, none of these ancient writings, Hebrew, Christian, or Islamic, contain the commandment "Thou shalt not use tobacco." Tobacco was introduced to the Old World from the Americas in the sixteenth century, and was unknown to the authors of ancient Hebrew, Christian, and Islamic writings. Nevertheless, many modern religions forbid tobacco use.

Before the dangers of tobacco were widely understood, it was acceptable for observant Jews to smoke. Today, however, many rabbis forbid smoking and condemn exposing others to secondhand smoke. One such rabbi quotes Maimonides, the greatest Jewish scholar of the Middle Ages, who wrote:

It is impossible to understand and perceive the knowledge of the Creator when one is sick; therefore a person must distance himself from things destructive to the body, and... conduct himself in those things that are strengthening and therapeutic.

About a quarter of the adherents of organized religion in the United States today are members of the Roman Catholic Church. Generally speaking, Roman Catholics view nicotine addiction as a medical problem—one that nevertheless may be a subject of prayer. The same is true of liberal Protestant denominations, including Episcopal, United Methodist, Presbyterian, and Congregationalist.

The large and fast-growing conservative Protestant denominations—Southern Baptist, Church of the Nazarene, Church of God, and Assemblies of God—have long maintained distinctive rules for the behavior of their members. Abstaining from tobacco use is one of these rules, along with abstaining from alcohol, illicit sex, gambling, and social dancing. Church members may shun a member who does not conform to the expected behavior. One teenage church member complained, "Since I started [smoking] people at the church [where] I go (adults and teens) won't talk to me!" Conservative Protestant colleges may require faculty, staff, and students to agree not to use tobacco.

Conservative Protestant churches often view smoking as a sin. Lecturing against smoking, one of their ministers says, "Every Christian is accountable to God for the condition of his body. As Christians, there should be no place in our lives for this evil habit." He quotes the New Testament verse which says, "I beseech you therefore, brethren, by the mercies of God, that ye present your bodies a living sacrifice, holy, acceptable unto God, which is your reasonable service."

Sects that are offshoots of Protestantism—the Latter-Day Saints (Mormons), Seventh-Day Adventists, Christian Scientists, and Jehovah's Witnesses—condemn tobacco use in different ways. Section 89 of the Mormon "Doctrine and Covenants," called the "Word of Wisdom," is considered by the church to be revelation from God given through the prophet Joseph Smith. The eighth verse of the Word of Wisdom says, "And, again, tobacco is not for the body, neither for the belly, and is not good for man…" Mormons are strongly discouraged from smoking and from drinking alcohol, coffee, or tea. A Mormon who smokes is not permitted to attend a Mormon temple. Attendance at a Mormon temple requires a card called a "recommend," stating that the bearer has lived up to all the agreements that he or she has made with the Mormon Church, and has demonstrated this to the satisfaction of certain church officials. It is estimated that only about one-fifth of Mormons have a recommend allowing them to attend a temple. Attendance and work at a temple is undertaken as a means of advancing to eventual deification. Thus, tobacco use would prevent a Mormon from becoming deified.

In the mid-1800s, the Seventh-Day Adventist denomination was formed. It now has hundreds of thousands of American members and millions of members in other countries. The General Conference of Seventh-Day Adventists has published a document called "Fundamental Beliefs" that constitutes "the church's understanding and expression of the teaching of Scripture." Section 21, "Christian Behavior," states:

For the Spirit to recreate in us the character of our Lord we involve ourselves only in those things which will produce Christlike purity, health, and joy in our lives... Since alcoholic beverages, tobacco, and the irresponsible use of drugs and narcotics are harmful to our bodies, we are to abstain from them.

A person seeking Adventist church membership must make a vow to abstain from "...the use, manufacture, or sale of tobacco in any of its forms for human consumption..." If a church member breaks this vow, he or she can be censured or lose church membership.

In 1879, Mary Baker Eddy founded the Church of Christ, Scientist, popularly known as Christian Science. In Christian Science, emphasis is placed on healing through spiritual means as an important element of Christianity. Christian Scientists believe that pure divine goodness underlies the scientific reality of existence. Thus, evils such as disease, death, and sin cannot be part of fundamental reality, but result from living apart from God. Christian Science teaches that prayer is the proper way to heal human ills. The Bible, plus Eddy's book, *Science and Health with Key to the Scriptures*, are Christian Science's sacred texts. In *Science and Health*, Eddy states that "...false appetites...yield to spirituality....The depraved appetite for alcoholic drinks, tobacco, tea, coffee, opium, is destroyed only by Mind's mastery of the body." Eddy's book is replete with testimonials from people who say that their nicotine addiction was overcome by a study of *Science and Health*.

Charles Taze Russell founded the Jehovah's Witnesses in the late 1800s. Witnesses often call their governing body, the Watchtower Bible and Tract Society, "God's visible organization." The Witnesses go door-to-door attempting to make converts. Once a person converts to their religion, the Witnesses exercise a good deal of control over his or her behavior. Witness elders are "overseers" who "have a large part in overseeing the cleanness of the congregation." The elders must "reprove and readjust wrongdoers" and "remove unrepentant wrongdoers." A document called "Pay Attention to Yourselves and to All the Flock" guides the elders in these duties. Behavior forbidden by this document includes "Misuse of tobacco or addictive drugs."

The Qur'an is the sacred text of Islam, considered by Muslims to contain God's revelations to the prophet Mohammed. Since Mohammed lived in the sixth and seventh centuries A.D., the Qur'an contains no mention of tobacco, which was then unknown except in the Americas. However, the Qur'an contains general prohibitions against harming a person's own health, or the health of others. As tobacco's dangers to health have become more and more certain, an increasing number of Islamic scholars have pronounced tobacco use forbidden to Muslims.

Hindus view tobacco use as a *vyasana*, which means a dependence that is not necessary to preserve health. A vyasana is inconsistent with a spiritual life. Moreover, smoking causes heart disease, and to Hindus the heart is an important symbol and a holy seat of God. Finally, Hindu scriptures say that "Doing good to others is an act of merit: harming others is a sinful act." Therefore, to Hindus, harming others by exposing them to secondhand smoke is a sin.

Buddhism emphasizes a path to freedom and enlightenment. Freedom, in Buddhist thought, means no dependence on anything, hence no addictions. Buddhists seek to abandon craving. Craving harms mental clarity, important to Buddhists. When a person is addicted to tobacco, he or she craves it, and is dependent on it. One Buddhist scholar says, "Doubtless the struggle against craving is hard…. If someone says that he has gotten over smoking, but he carries cigars about him for the sake of a test, then he has not yet fully abandoned craving." Another Buddhist scholar says that a person should "avoid misusing [the body] as an instrument only for pleasure. We should be very careful not to form habits which are injurious to the body, such as smoking…"

170 Smokers are less desirable as dates and potential mates.

Nonsmokers, who outnumber smokers almost four to one in the United States, nearly always prefer not to date or marry smokers. This restricts a smoker's choice of dates and potential mates.

Nonsmokers don't want to be exposed to secondhand smoke on a date, either from their companion or from sitting in the smoking section of a restaurant or other public place. When a smoker who smokes in his or her apartment invites a date in, the apartment will smell of stale tobacco smoke—a definite turnoff to a nonsmoker. An automobile that smells of tobacco smoke is also a turnoff.

And smoking makes both men and women physically unattractive in a variety of ways. Hair, clothing, and breath smell of smoke. Teeth, fingers, and fingernails may be stained. Older smokers usually have more wrinkles and poorer skin. Cigarette cough and sputum production are unattractive.

A nonsmoker who is looking for a marriage partner usually won't want to waste time dating smokers. If you are a woman who smokes, most male non-smokers—who usually are more successful breadwinners than male smokers— won't want to marry you. Smokers are poor marriage prospects because they have an expensive addiction that may result in chronic ill health and early death. And the babies of a woman who smokes are less likely to be healthy. Moreover, nonsmokers don't want a lifetime of breathing secondhand smoke generated by a smoking mate. Some nonsmokers have religious beliefs that prevent them from considering a smoker as a life partner. And some nonsmokers may view smokers as lacking in character and therefore not acceptable as potential mates.

This preference for nonsmokers is reflected in newspaper and internet classified ads for dates and potential mates. A large percentage of ads specify that the person is looking for a nonsmoker, and many people begin by describing themselves as nonsmokers—evidently perceiving this as even more important than "well-educated," "handsome," "athletic," and the like.

Dating service questionnaires almost always ask about the smoking status of the person applying, as well as his or her preference as to the smoking status of the person he or she is seeking. Rarely does anyone say they are seeking a smoker, and the few who do are almost always smokers themselves.

Family Relationships

171 **Smoking can strain or even disrupt your marriage. People who smoke are more likely to divorce than those who don't.**

Marriage counselors advise nonsmokers to marry nonsmokers. Marriages in which one spouse smokes and the other does not can be severely strained. When two smokers marry, dissension can arise if one quits smoking and the other does not.

A nonsmoking spouse may come to resent exposure to cigarette smoke as more and more evidence piles up on the dangers of secondhand smoke. One wife says, "When we were first married 40 years ago, I didn't mind his smoking. Now that we are in our 70s, I have respiratory problems as well as eye problems, and the smoke is very irritating. He refuses to believe that secondhand smoke is injurious to others. We rarely watch television together, as I leave the room when he lights up. I miss the closeness we once had."

A nonsmoking spouse may want to enjoy a meal in the nonsmoking section of a restaurant, or sit in the nonsmoking area in an airport, train, or other public place, while the smoking spouse wants to sit in the smoking section. This can cause resentment, dissension, or outright fights. One man who insisted on having his meal in a restaurant's nonsmoking section said he was offended when, halfway through dinner, his wife left him to light up a cigarette in the bar.

A nonsmoking parent may worry about exposing the children to a spouse's cigarette smoke. This can be a major source of stress and anxiety. The wife of a man who smokes two and a half packs a day says, "Our six-year-old has allergy problems, and our four-year-old wakes up coughing. I love the guy, but if I could live my life over, I would never marry a smoker."

A spouse's smoking can interfere with the couple's sex life. Smoking is a major risk factor for atherosclerosis, one of the most common physical conditions underlying male impotence. Men who smoke cigarettes are much more likely to become impotent than nonsmokers, and even young husbands are at risk. One study showed that, in men 31 to 49 years of age, the rate of impotence among the smokers was 50 percent higher than among the nonsmokers. Moreover, Viagra, a drug designed to counteract impotence, is not as effective in smokers.

A spouse's smoking can make him or her so unattractive to the other spouse that it interferes with their sex life. One wife says, "Mike smells like his stinking cigarettes all the time. The odor is repulsive to me and a real turn-off. I can hardly stand for him to touch me. He has chosen to give up closeness and intimacy rather than give up smoking."

Nonsmoking spouses often resent the strain on family finances, especially if the family is on a tight budget. Arguments arise over the amount of money being spent on cigarettes, higher insurance premiums, more doctors' bills, and replacing clothing and furniture that have cigarette burns. A nonsmoking spouse who feels he or she is making financial sacrifices so that the other can smoke may be unpleasant to live with.

The additional housework caused by smoking is a problem in some marriages. Conflict is especially likely if the nonsmoking spouse is the housekeeper. Overflowing ashtrays, smoke stains on the walls and ceilings, cigarette butts littering the yard, drapes that smell of smoke—all these make housekeeping more difficult. Cigarette smoke permeates clothing, so the amount of laundry may be increased. Women, who are the housekeepers in most marriages, often work outside the home as well. If a working wife has children, her burden is even heavier. The additional housework caused by a spouse's smoking could create an intolerable situation.

Anyone trying to quit smoking ordinarily finds quitting more difficult if his or her spouse smokes. Constantly seeing someone else smoking, and smelling cigarette smoke, increases the temptation to relapse. This can cause resentment on the part of the spouse who is trying to quit.

On the other hand, the spouse who continues to smoke may resent being told to go outside to smoke, or being heckled to quit smoking. One smoker whose husband had quit smoking said, "My husband nagged me for six months to quit after he did. That made me more determined than ever to keep smoking. For reasons that are still unclear to me, he decided on his own to stop nagging and criticizing." She finally decided to quit smoking for herself. Her husband was her major support. This outcome undoubtedly strengthened the marriage.

Some people go to extreme lengths to get a spouse to quit smoking. One man, married 47 years, said he had argued for years with his wife about her smoking. Finally, he rented a billboard on a busy highway that read, "Phyllis J. S____. Stop Your Smoking! We love you. From your family and friends." He drove her past the billboard, which he said upset her. Whether or not she stopped smoking is unknown.

Another man sued his wife to get her to stop smoking. He claimed in his complaint to the court that his wife was violating the federal Clean Air Act. Before the court had made a decision, his wife agreed to stop smoking and he asked that the lawsuit be dismissed.

Unfortunately, many marital disputes over smoking do not end as happily. A study at the University of Minnesota found that adults who smoke are 53 percent more likely to divorce than those who don't smoke. Marriage counselors recommend joint counseling when spouses are in conflict over smoking.

172 If you smoke, family members may worry about your health. In many families, strain and tension ensue when worried family members try to convince a smoker to quit.

Smoking often causes a great deal of worry to a smoker's family members. They worry about the smoker's health, which they may see deteriorating. A smoker's husband or wife may worry that the smoker will die early. Smokers have died in their 30s or 40s from lung cancer, heart disease, and other smoking-related illnesses. Thus, cigarettes have widowed many spouses prematurely, robbing them of the deceased spouse's support and companionship. Widowed spouses have been left without financial support. Some have been left to raise children alone.

Parents worry when their children smoke. A nonsmoker said, "I have been lecturing, nagging and clipping articles and statistics in an effort to educate those I love. My wife has been smoking since she was 15. Even more upsetting, four of our seven children are hooked." The child of a parent who smokes is much more likely to take up smoking. When a child takes up smoking, the parent who smokes may feel guilty, in addition to being worried about the child's health.

Children worry when their parents smoke. One woman said, "My mother is on a respirator because of severe lung damage. She has asthma and smoked cigarettes for 50 years. Now she has emphysema and pneumonia. For years the family asked her to quit smoking, but it was something she couldn't—or didn't want to—do."

A man related his story: "For years as I was growing up, my mother and I tried everything we knew to get my father to quit smoking, but despite our best efforts, he could not break his habit. Little by little over the years I could see how smoking robbed him of his health. His visits to the doctor and then the hospital became more frequent, and his list of medications grew."

Even young children—who learn in school and youth groups, and from sports coaches and television, about the dangers of smoking—worry about the health of parents who smoke. They fear that they may become orphans. Many confront their parents, asking, "Why are you smoking when you know it could kill you?" Some post "No Smoking" signs, or skull-and-crossbones posters, around the house. Some enterprising kids hide or destroy their parents' cigarettes.

One 12-year-old ran away from home to protest his parents' smoking.

Children sometimes succeed in getting their parents to stop smoking. A pre-teen son and daughter waged a relentless war against their parents' smoking and finally won. Their parents promised to quit if they both promised never to start. But in many families the children's war against their parents' smoking produces strain and tension, pitting parent against child.

Child-rearing authorities have addressed parent-child conflicts over parental smoking. One authority says, "If a parent does something that really scares a child, and won't stop when he or she protests, it tells the child that the parent doesn't care how the child feels. The role of the parent is to nurture and protect, not to do something the child equates with being made an orphan." One mother, who understood this, quit smoking after she had a nightmare in which she was dying of lung cancer while her two-year-old son stood by her bed crying, "Don't leave me, Mommy!" This mother said, "If you can't quit for yourself, quit for those who love you."

173 Someone who dies of a smoking-related illness may leave behind loved ones whose grief is increased by the thought that the death could have been prevented.

Smoking is estimated to cause about 440,000 deaths each year in the United States. These smokers leave behind an enormous number of survivors. The grief of these survivors is often increased by the thought that the smoker's death could have been prevented.

One woman says, "My mother passed away when she was only 65 years old. She had smoked for decades. She got emphysema that killed her. I don't have a mother now and my children don't have a grandma. Smokers, please think about the pain and suffering you can cause your family by continuing to smoke."

Many smokers who die from smoking-related illnesses leave a spouse without companionship and support. A widow said, "My husband was only 58 when he died of congestive heart failure and chronic obstructive pulmonary disease aggravated by cigarette smoking. We had been married 40 years, and I will always wonder how many years his life was shortened by smoking."

Smoking is often called "slow suicide." Survivors of a person who dies of a smoking-related illness may suffer guilt similar to that of a suicide's survivors. The survivors may feel that they are somehow responsible, that they could have prevented the death if only they had been more diligent, pressed harder, done *something* to make the smoker quit.

One son says, "My dad died from lung cancer caused by his smoking. If only I had tried harder, maybe I could have persuaded him to quit before it was too late. Instead, I just bought into his argument that it was his business whether to smoke or not."

A woman whose mother died of lung cancer said people asked her, "Was your mother a smoker?" This added to the daughter's grief by "making it sound like her death was justified." Sparing your loved ones from the added grief that attends a smoking-related death is an excellent reason to quit smoking.

174 Family anger, resentment, embarrassment, and disappointment with family members who smoke are important reasons to avoid tobacco.

Smokers cause many problems for other family members, including exposure to secondhand smoke, a greatly increased risk of fire, and the burden of caring for a disabled smoker with a smoking-related illness. As a result, some family members feel anger and resentment toward the smoker. Others feel embarrassment or disappointment.

One man recalled a Christmas at his mother's house where two of his cousins, his brother, and his sister-in-law were smoking. "I got so angry when I saw that they were exposing my two-year-old son to their smoke. I told them that if they wanted to smoke, they had to do it in the garage. My brother objected, but finally all four of them retreated to the garage, where they spent most of Christmas day."

A wife, whose mother-in-law lived with her and her husband, said her mother-in-law had tried for years to hide her smoking from them. Finally, lung disease caused by smoking landed the mother-in-law in the intensive care unit of a hospital. When she came back to their home, she was housebound and hooked to an oxygen tank. The wife reports that her husband "bitterly resents the hell she has put us all through. He is very impatient with his mother, and it has ruined their relationship."

A man whose wife pretended to be a nonsmoker said to her, "I'm embarrassed by this. I suspect our family and friends know because of the smell, the cough, and all the other signs. Whenever we meet after being apart and I smell the smoke on your breath, in your clothes and in your hair, I feel a stab of disappointment."

Family anger, resentment, embarrassment, and disappointment are important reasons to quit smoking. If you quit smoking, you'll most likely find that your family members are relieved, especially if you quit before smoking has ruined your health.

175 If you smoke, you may be at a disadvantage in a child custody or visitation dispute. And you may be unable to adopt a child or become a foster parent.

Millions of minor children are the subjects of legal disputes over their custody, or over a parent's right to visit them, usually as a result of divorce proceedings. Judges in family courts decide these cases based on what appears to be in the best interest of the child. They take many factors into consideration, including a parent's use of alcohol or drugs. In the 1980s, judges also began taking into account the health risk to children from secondhand smoke.

Usually, the judge first orders the parent to refrain from smoking around the child. If the parent disobeys the judge's order, the parent may lose custody. In a California case, for example, an eight-year-old girl with asthma was removed from her mother's custody and placed with her grandmother when the mother continued to violate a court order forbidding her to smoke around the child.

Parental smoking also affects visitation rights:

■ A judge in a Pennsylvania case ordered a father to cease smoking in his home at least 48 hours before his children arrived to visit.

■ A Louisiana court reduced a father's visitation rights because his smoking made his child's bronchial illness worse.

■ At a child's request, a New York judge ordered the child's mother not to smoke in her apartment or car, on penalty of losing visitation rights.

■ An Ohio judge learned that both parents in a custody and visitation case were smoking in their homes. On his own initiative, the judge issued an order forbidding them to smoke in the presence of the child. In his decision, this judge wrote, "A family court that fails to issue court orders restraining persons from smoking in the presence of children under its jurisdiction is failing the children whom the law has entrusted to its care."

Even in an intact marriage, it is possible for parents to lose custody if they willfully expose the child to secondhand smoke. Under child abuse and neglect laws, physicians, school nurses, and teachers may have a legal duty to file a complaint when they become aware of a child whose parents are significantly endangering his health by exposing him to secondhand smoke. Children with asthma, allergies, or sinusitis are in special need of such protection, because secondhand smoke exposure can trigger attacks of these illnesses. If parents violate a court order to stop smoking around a child, they could lose custody.

If you smoke, you may have trouble adopting a child. Adoption agencies prefer nonsmokers, and may refuse to place a child in a home where one of the potential parents smokes. This is not an unreasonable rule, because it would probably be impossible to make certain that the adopted child was not exposed to secondhand smoke. In addition, children whose parents smoke are more likely to become smokers themselves.

Some states and counties are protecting foster children from secondhand smoke. The state is responsible for foster children, and may forbid smoking in the home or car when a foster child is present. John F. Banzhaf, III, Executive Director and Chief Counsel for Action on Smoking and Health (ASH) has filed a Foster Care Petition pointing out that foster care agencies have "a moral—as well as a legal—obligation to protect foster children, who are defenseless wards of the state, from easily preventable and readily foreseeable harm [from secondhand tobacco smoke]." You can read this petition on the ash.org website.

Moreover, some of these protections for foster children are being extended to all children in some states. In California, smoking in a car can result in a $100 fine if anyone younger than 18 is present. In Maine, a driver can be stopped and penalized for allowing anyone to smoke in the vehicle if a person under 16 is a passenger.

176 Long-term smokers often suffer extended disabilities from smoking-related illnesses, thus exposing family members to the stress of caregiving.

There is a better than 50 percent chance that an American will be called on, at some point in life, to become the primary caregiver for an aging or ailing family member. Only ten to

20 percent of people who require care are in nursing homes. Most are cared for at home, where the caregiver may supervise in-home assistance, but usually provides the care personally.

Caregivers perform such tasks as feeding, lifting, bathing, grooming, toileting, and dressing the disabled person. Caregivers also give medications, shop for groceries, provide transportation, and do household chores. Caregiving is sometimes a round-the-clock job, with the needs of the disabled person interrupting the caregiver's sleep. Most caregivers have little time for themselves. Navigating a complex healthcare system can add to the caregiver's burden, as can worrying about unpaid medical expenses. The caregiver's relationships with other family members— spouse, children, or siblings—may become strained.

The need to care for a parent usually arises when the lives of adult children are most stressful, with children and jobs that also require their energies. On the other hand, many caregivers, particularly spouses of disabled people, are themselves elderly. Thirty-eight percent of caregivers are over 50 years old. About 72 percent of caregivers are women—the wives, daughters, sisters, or daughters-in-law of those who need care.

Modern medicine keeps many chronically disabled people alive for extended periods of time. Nursing homes are expensive—the average cost is over $60,000 a year. The Medicaid system in the United States pays for care of the chronically disabled in nursing homes after they have used up ("spent down") their own money. But a majority of caregivers maintain a disabled spouse, parent, or sibling at home.

A caregiver may feel guilty about putting an ailing family member into a nursing home, or fear (rightly in some instances) that a nursing home will not provide good care. Often, the disabled person resists being put into a nursing home. Unfortunately, there is little government financial assistance for people who provide home care.

The greatest reward for a caregiver is the feeling that a family member is being well cared for and is happier at home. But caregivers have more high blood pressure, infectious diseases, and heart disease than the general population. They also have a greater risk of early death. Research suggests that the chronic stress of caregiving may do lasting harm to the immune system. Medical professionals call this "caregiver syndrome."

Caregiving can result in isolation, fatigue, and stress, which in turn can lead to feelings of anger, resentment, guilt, and depression. A woman who took care of her husband for 23 years, after he had a first heart attack at age 38, said she became "an extension of the illness." She inwardly raged at her loss of freedom, intimacy, and partnership, yet believed that her feelings were wrong and selfish.

A wife with three teenaged sons is also responsible for helping three elderly parents. Her mother, who is legally blind, lives with her. Her father is in a nursing home, and her mother-in-law is sometimes bedridden with arthritis. She says, "I always feel guilty that I don't do enough. I don't go to the nursing home enough. I don't help my mother-in-law enough."

Most people dread becoming a burden to others. A loss of independence and dignity is hard on anyone. A chronically disabled person may become depressed, angry, or even abusive, adding to the caregiver's burdens.

Although some illnesses are unavoidable, if you take good care of your health you are far less likely to have an extended disability. Long-term smokers are at much greater risk than nonsmokers of extended disabilities from cancer, emphysema, heart disease, stroke, peripheral artery disease, macular degeneration, or other ailments. Maintaining your independence for as long as possible, thus sparing family members from the stress of extended caregiving, is a good reason to avoid tobacco.

177 If you smoke, you may perceive yourself as weak-willed and lacking self-control. Your family may perceive you that way, too. But they will be proud of you if you quit smoking.

Most people know that conquering an addiction to nicotine is difficult, and have respect for someone who succeeds. If you quit smoking, your self-esteem will get a major boost from the congratulations of family members.

Many smokers have low self-esteem because they perceive themselves as weak-willed and lacking self-control. They may feel that other people perceive them that way, too. Quitting proves to themselves and to others that this is not true. Even family members who themselves smoke may be supportive and proud of a person who has quit smoking.

You will probably be pleasantly surprised by how eager your family is to support your effort to quit. So declare your intention and tell the people who care about you how they can help. If missing that last cigarette before bedtime is the worst obstacle for you, your daughter might volunteer to read you her favorite bedtime story until you fall asleep. If the craving for that first morning cigarette with your coffee is the hardest time for you, your husband might serve you breakfast in bed. Not only will your family love and respect you for making their lives easier and less stressful, they will be proud of you for conquering your addiction and proud of themselves for helping.

Social and Professional Relationships

178 A smoker is a poor role model who may influence others to smoke.

An important reason not to smoke is that if you smoke you may influence other people to smoke. Recent studies show that social groups may start smoking en masse—groups of teenaged friends, for example. But if you quit smoking you may influence others to quit. Social groups also tend to quit smoking en masse.

Peer pressure affects adults as well as teenagers. A study by the federal Centers for Disease Control found that the greatest decline in the number of adult smokers has been among people with the highest levels of education. One of the researchers said, "It has nothing to do with intelligence, but with social milieu....Social pressure is what convinces a lot of people to stop smoking." Another study found that married couples tend to mimic each other in lowering health risk factors, including smoking. Thus, if one spouse quits smoking, the other is also more likely to quit.

If you are a parent who smokes, your child is much more likely to smoke. Antismoking lectures from a parent who smokes are likely to fall on deaf ears. Seventy-five percent of teenagers who smoke have at least one parent who smokes.

Nicotine addiction often repeats itself in successive generations of a family.

However, when a parent quits smoking it sends a powerful message to his or her children. Moreover, the younger a child is when the parent quits, the more influence quitting will have. Some children begin smoking as early as fourth grade, so don't think you can wait to quit until your child is a teenager.

During the teenage years, the parents' influence decreases and the influence of the child's peer group increases. If smoking is thought to be "cool" among a teenager's peer group, the chances are greater that the teenager will smoke. One teenager said, "A lot of kids who smoke don't want to smoke, but it's the influence of their friends that keeps them going." A child whose friends are nonsmokers is much less likely to smoke. One study of 9,965 teenagers found that 50 percent of teenagers with friends who smoked were smokers themselves, while only three percent of teenagers with friends who didn't smoke had taken up smoking. This study also found that older brothers and sisters who smoked were an especially bad influence on their younger siblings.

Movie and television stars, professional ballplayers, rock stars, fashion models, and other celebrities serve as role models for millions of people. Celebrities who smoke may make smoking appear glamorous and exciting, especially to children and teenagers. One study of 632 teenagers found that teens whose favorite celebrity smoked were three times more likely to smoke than teens whose favorite celebrity did not smoke.

Humor columnist Bill Hall wrote, "It wouldn't exactly be accurate to say that I blame Humphrey Bogart for all the years I spent smoking cigarettes. It would be more accurate to say that I blame Humphrey Bogart, John Wayne, my father, Bette Davis, my mother, Edward R. Murrow, several uncles and aunts, William Holden, dozens of major league baseball players, Frank Sinatra, the dirty rotten lying tobacco company executives, and myself, of course, especially myself." Hall says that he saw the light and quit smoking by the time he was 40.

Health activists have long been pressuring the Motion Picture Association of America to take smoking into account, along with violence, nudity, language, drug abuse, and other elements, when assigning a rating to a movie. In 2007, the Association agreed to consider smoking when assigning ratings. But this falls short of what the health activists would like—an R rating (Restricted—under 17 not admitted without a parent) for any movie where actors smoke.

Actors who smoke in real life, as well as in the movies, often develop serious smoking-related illnesses. Then they may deeply regret the influence that their on-screen smoking had on their audiences. Jack Klugman, an actor who got cancer of the larynx as a result of 40 years of smoking, is now an anti-smoking activist who wrote the Foreword to this book. Klugman says that John Garfield and other movie heroes who smoked on screen influenced him to begin smoking. He regrets his own on-screen smoking and says, "Now that we know how terrible smoking is and how terrible it is for children to emulate this behavior, there is no reason for smoking on screen—unless you're doing a story about someone affected by smoking."

Screenwriter Joe Eszterhas, who developed throat cancer after a lifetime of smoking, says, "Smoking was an integral part of many of my screenplays.... Smoking, I once believed, was every person's right...I don't think smoking is every person's right anymore. I think smoking should be as illegal as heroin.... I have been an accomplice in the murders of untold numbers of human beings." Celebrities have a special moral obligation not to influence children and teenagers to begin smoking.

Teachers, coaches, physicians, and nurses also have a special moral obligation not to influence others to smoke. One man said, "When I began teaching school, I knew I had to quit smoking because I couldn't continue to smoke and tell my students it was bad for them." Few doctors smoke, but those who do provide an especially bad example for patients, who may think that if their doctor smokes there must be nothing wrong with it.

179 Smoking can strain friendships in many ways and sometimes costs the smoker a valued friend.

Family and romantic relationships aren't the only ones strained—sometimes beyond repair—by smoking. Smoking causes problems among friends, too.

Today, more than ever, smokers make friends with others who smoke. This is natural because, increasingly, smokers are thrown together in ever smaller and more segregated spaces. With other smokers as friends, a smoker feels that he is not being judged for his smoking and for exposing others to secondhand smoke. But friendships built around smoking often face insurmountable problems when one of the friends decides to quit.

Someone who decides to quit smoking may be discouraged from doing so by smoking buddies who don't want to lose his companionship. Abandoning these friends is justifiable because the peril posed by tobacco is literally a matter of life and death. And when you quit smoking you will have a much larger number of people from which to choose new friends—the nonsmokers.

Many people who have never smoked have friends who do and, here again, smoking often puts a strain on the friendship. In one case, eight friends, all of whom worked at the same plant, decided to celebrate one friend's birthday at a restaurant. The headwaiter asked, "Smoking or nonsmoking?" One member of the group said, "Nonsmoking, please." Another spoke up, "Wait a minute! Three of us are smokers." The group ended up sitting in the smoking section, where the smokers chain-smoked for two hours, spoiling the meal for the nonsmokers and straining the group's friendships.

Many people don't allow smoking in their homes or cars, and may stop inviting their friends who smoke in an effort to avoid a confrontation. Nonsmokers frequently don't want to visit a friend who smokes in his house—much less eat dinner there. The smell of stale tobacco smoke (often unnoticeable to the smoker who lives there) can be obnoxious to a nonsmoker. In addition, most nonsmokers these days know that exposure to secondhand smoke can compromise health.

For example, two women, one a smoker, met at an outdoor playground where their two preschool children played. The women found that they had a great deal in common and formed a friendship. Since they were outdoors, the nonsmoker wasn't concerned about exposure to her new friend's secondhand smoke. But when the smoker invited the nonsmoker's daughter to her home to play with her son, the nonsmoker asked if she smoked in the house. When the smoker said, "Yes," the nonsmoker said she couldn't let her daughter be exposed to secondhand smoke. That ended their friendship.

180 The smell of secondhand smoke is an irresistible temptation to many former smokers. To keep from relapsing, they may have to avoid friends who smoke or change jobs.

Most smokers find it difficult to quit smoking, and once they have quit they must be on guard against relapsing. Many former smokers say that they get a powerful urge to smoke whenever they smell secondhand tobacco smoke. A person making a real effort to quit won't be able to accompany smoking friends to smoky bars, sit with them in the smoking sections of restaurants, or even be around them at all without being tempted to resume smoking. The harsh reality is that a former smoker may have to stop spending time with friends who smoke. And it may be necessary for him to change jobs in order to have a smoke-free workplace.

The problem of avoiding secondhand smoke is more difficult when it is a spouse or other family member who smokes. Smokers who have a family member who has quit smoking have another reason to "take it outside" instead of smoking in the house.

181 Employees who don't smoke often resent the extra burdens placed on them by coworkers who do.

Bad feelings between employees who smoke and those who don't are rampant in many companies. Smokers take 50 percent more sick leave, often creating a heavier workload for other employees. In workplaces where smokers must leave the premises to smoke, frequent smoking breaks take smokers away from the job, in many cases leaving other employees to cover for them. Where smokers are allowed to smoke on the job, the amount of time that smoking occupies is obvious to the nonsmokers, who may resent what they see as other employees wasting time.

Job accidents are another source of tension between smokers and nonsmokers. Even smokers who don't smoke on the job have more accidents than nonsmokers—accidents that may result in injury to other employees. And people who do smoke on the job sometimes ignite workplace fires that cause injuries, job interruption, or even destruction of the employer's business.

Yet another common cause of tension between smoking and nonsmoking employees is an increase in health insurance cost due to smoking-related illnesses. Most people obtain health insurance through employer group plans. Often the employees pay part or all of the premiums for their group health insurance. Those premiums are based on the health of the group as a whole, so groups of employees with higher rates of illness pay higher premiums. Nonsmoking employees may resent paying the higher cost of group health insurance that results from smoking-related illnesses.

Although most employers now restrict or ban smoking in the workplace, some employers still do not. Secondhand smoke exposure usually causes discomfort to nonsmokers, irritating their eyes, noses, and throats. The World Health Organization says, "In premises without efficient ventilation, working in a cloud of blue smoke can become a real torment [causing] tension and ill humor..." Moreover, many nonsmokers are concerned about the serious adverse effects on their health from secondhand smoke, leading to tensions among coworkers.

In some workplaces, nonsmoking employees have pressured management to eliminate smoking on the job. In one instance, the employer had restricted smoking to the cafeteria and lounges. Several hundred nonsmoking employees signed a petition asking management to ban smoking on company premises, pointing out that allowing it in the cafeteria and lounges concentrated the smoke there and made those places unendurable to nonsmokers. Smoking employees signed a counter-petition, complaining that smoking outdoors in a climate that sometimes dipped below zero in the winter would cause them considerable hardship. Management resolved the dispute by converting one lounge to a smoking room that had large fans ventilating the smoke to the outdoors, while smoking was banned elsewhere on company premises. This far-sighted company also decided to pay for employee stop-smoking clinics to help those smokers who wanted to quit. Nevertheless, tensions between nonsmokers and smokers, from what became known as "The Great Smoking War," continued for some time.

182 Smokers frustrate doctors and dentists, some of whom refuse to treat them.

In an ideal relationship between a doctor and a patient, the doctor educates the patient about taking care of his or her health, and the patient follows the doctor's advice. Patients frustrate doctors when they expect a doctor to "fix" every ailment, but refuse to take responsibility for their own health. One doctor says that she does not feel that "it is the job of primary-care physicians to prevent and control lifestyle-related illnesses such as those associated with obesity and smoking." She goes on to say, "We are all responsible for the decisions we make regarding risk-taking behaviors, and doctors suffer the frustration of educating and working with patients for whom we care deeply but cannot help because they cannot or will not help themselves." Although most doctors feel that they have a duty to care for such people, some refuse to do so. The American Medical Association Code of Ethics leaves doctors free to choose whom they will treat, as long as they don't discriminate on the basis of race, color, or creed, or refuse to give emergency treatment.

Some doctors refuse to treat smokers. One doctor states that smokers are not meeting their responsibilities, and he will not treat them unless they quit. He argues that smokers knowingly harm their health while making nonsmokers foot the bill through higher insurance premiums, Medicare, and Medicaid.

Another doctor says he will only accept patients who smoke if they come to him to be treated for nicotine addiction. Yet another doctor who won't treat smokers says that doctors need to come down hard on patients with unhealthy behaviors that contribute to huge health care costs. And, as one doctor pointed out:

If you make no serious effort to stop smoking, eat a healthy diet, get some exercise, and reduce stress, even the most dedicated doctor may well begin to think of time spent with you as time wasted.

Dentists, too, get frustrated with patients who smoke. Smokers have more cavities, more gum disease, and more tooth loss than nonsmokers. Periodontal surgery and tooth implants are more likely to fail, and other dental treatments are less likely to be successful. One dentist refuses to work on any patient who smokes unless a dental hygienist has just cleaned that patient's teeth. Then, while the patient is in the chair with a mouth full of cotton balls, the dentist gives the patient a nonstop lecture on the harm that smoking is doing to his or her dental health.

ECONOMIC COSTS

Direct Costs of Smoking

183 **Cigarettes are costly and almost certain to become more so. A person who smokes heavily may see two to three hundred dollars a month go up in smoke.**

The decision to smoke is costly. A young person who avoids tobacco has a far better chance of lifelong financial health than one who becomes addicted. One writer pointed out that "smoking is hazardous to your wealth." The cost of cigarettes is only the beginning, but it is substantial.

The retail price of cigarettes is determined by several elements:

- The costs of manufacturing, advertising, and distributing cigarettes.

- The cost to the major tobacco companies of their estimated $246 billion settlement with the states to help defray Medicaid expenses for smoking-related illnesses.

- The profit margins of the tobacco companies, wholesalers, and retailers.

- Taxes—federal excise tax, state and local cigarette taxes, and state and local sales taxes. Every state and many cities set their own cigarette and sales taxes, which vary greatly.

Cigarette prices also vary greatly. In 2008, the average retail price across the country of a pack of cigarettes was between $4 and $5. But in some places, such as New York City, they sold for $8 to $9 a pack. Discount cigarettes bought over the internet by the carton cost between $1 and $2 a pack, before taxes. These internet sales of cigarettes, which have often been untaxed, are more likely to be taxed in the future, due largely to the efforts of Action on Smoking and Health (ASH), a national anti-smoking and nonsmokers' rights organization.

Although cigarettes are cheaper if bought by the carton, it is estimated that 60 percent of cigarettes are bought by the pack, often at convenience stores. This is the most expensive way to buy cigarettes, but many smokers don't have the cash to buy them in more economical ways. Thus, the poorest smokers usually pay the most for their cigarettes. And many smokers tell themselves that every pack is the last one, and therefore don't purchase cigarettes by the carton.

A person who smokes heavily can easily see several hundred dollars go up in smoke every month. Numerous government agencies and private analysts have done estimates showing how much money can be earned by a person who quits smoking and invests what he or she would have spent on cigarettes. For instance, suppose on January 1, 2008, a 25-year-old pack-a-day smoker quits smoking. In 2008, he would have spent $1,679 if he had paid the average price of $4.60 a pack for cigarettes. But the price of cigarettes will almost certainly continue to increase. Cigarette prices rise with inflation and may exceed inflation if the tobacco companies lose additional lawsuits or enter into more settlements. Moreover, there is a trend toward higher cigarette taxes. For example, in April 2009, federal excise taxes on cigarettes increased from 39 cents to $1.01 per pack. Many cash-strapped states are considering cigarette tax increases. Therefore, it is reasonable to assume that cigarette prices will increase at least five percent a year. Thus, over 40 years, the cumulative amount that our former smoker would have spent on cigarettes approximates $203,000.

Now, suppose that, at the end of each year, our former smoker invests the money not spent on cigarettes in a qualified retirement plan. Assuming a six percent compounded annual investment return over 40 years, at age 65 his retirement fund would approximate $578,000. Moreover, he would more likely be alive to enjoy the money, and have a bonus of better health as well.

184 The annual medical costs of treating smoking-related illnesses are estimated to equal six to eight percent of all medical care costs.

Treating smoking-related illnesses costs tens of billions of dollars each year in the United States. These costs are estimated to equal six to eight percent of all medical care costs. Smokers themselves directly bear part of this expense in the form of increased health insurance premiums, insurance deductibles, coinsurance payments, and various unreimbursed costs. Society as a whole bears part of the cost in the form of Medicare and Medicaid payments, and increased insurance costs for government employees who smoke. Employers with group health plans (and employees who pay part or all of the premiums for some of these plans) also bear part of the cost. The employers' costs may be passed on to consumers.

The argument has been made that smoking does not actually increase medical care costs as a whole because smokers die younger than nonsmokers. The costs of medical care for nonsmokers during their extra years of life arguably cancel out the costs of treating preventable, smoking-related illnesses. Even if true, it cannot be comforting to the individual smoker to think that early death may cancel out the costs of treating his or her smoking-related illnesses. Wouldn't you would opt for a long life, and for medical care dollars to be spent taking care of you when you are old? If you would, then don't smoke.

185 If you smoke you will pay more for the types of insurance that are vital to most people.

Insurance companies have long known that the risk of early death, illness, injury, disability, house fires, and vehicle crashes is greater for smokers than for nonsmokers. Therefore, the types of insurance vital for most people—including life, health, disability income, long-term care, homeowners, and automobile insurance—usually cost smokers more. If smokers were not required to pay more for these types of insurance, then insureds who don't smoke would have their premiums increased to cover the increased risk caused by the smokers. This would not be fair.

The difference in life insurance premium rates for smokers versus nonsmokers can be substantial. For example, to insure the life of a healthy 35-year-old male for $250,000 under a 20-year-term policy, one well-known life insurance company charges a nonsmoker an annual premium of $203, but charges a smoker $738. The same policy issued to a healthy 61-year-old male has an annual premium of $2,078 for a nonsmoker, but $6,308 for a smoker. An applicant who is a heavy smoker—for example, someone who smokes 40 or more cigarettes a day—might receive a substandard rating, in addition to the higher smoker premium rate. A substandard rating will increase the premium rate even more. Moreover, many smokers have smoking-related diseases that result in a premium higher than the regular smoker premium, or that cause them to be uninsurable. A life insurance company will not issue any policy on the life of a person who is uninsurable.

Life insurance protects dependents against financial hardship in the event of the insured person's death. Most life policies are individual insurance, sold directly to the insured person. When you apply, one of the questions on the application deals with tobacco use. Typically, it asks, "Have you used any type of tobacco within the last three years?" The insurance company also may require a urine test to check for signs of tobacco use. Sometimes applicants give false answers to the question about tobacco use. But if, after the insured's death, the insurer discovers the truth from the insured's medical files or death certificate, the policy might be declared void, in which case no death benefit will be paid.

Health insurance pays for doctor, hospital, and other medically necessary services. Unlike life insurance, most health insurance in the United States is provided through employer group health plans. These plans cover the employees' dependents, as well as the employees themselves. Some employers require employees who smoke (or whose dependents smoke) to pay an extra amount for their health insurance, because having smokers in the group increases the cost of the group plan. For example, the amount paid for a 35-year-old nonsmoker is about three-fourths that for a 35-year-old who smokes. The difference is even greater at older ages. The amount paid for a 55-year-old nonsmoker is less than half that for a smoker. One insurance expert advises, "Cash-crunched employers should pay only the nonsmoker part of the cost [and require the smoker to pay the difference]." Individual health insurance policies, sold directly to people not covered by group plans, cost smokers more than nonsmokers.

Disability income insurance protects against the loss of income when an insured person becomes disabled and is unable to work. Only a minority of employers have group disability income plans covering their employees. A worker who lacks group disability income coverage can purchase an individual policy. As with life and health insurance, disability income insurance is sold using smoker and nonsmoker rates.

Long-term-care insurance can protect a family from financial ruin if the insured needs skilled nursing or custodial care for an extended period of time. The cost of long-term care can be substantial, averaging over $60,000 a year. And some older people with significant assets may want to protect those assets for a spouse or heirs by purchasing long-term-care insurance. Although Medicaid pays for the nursing home care of people who have few or no assets, some nursing homes do not accept Medicaid recipients. Therefore, some people purchase long-term-care insurance to avoid the limited nursing home options available to Medicaid recipients. Applicants for long-term-care insurance are usually over 55. They must be healthy when they apply or the insurer will not issue a policy. Insurers take smoking into consideration, asking questions such as, "Have you used any tobacco in the last 24 months?" As with other types of insurance, smokers pay more.

Homeowners' insurance protects against loss from fire, burglary, and other types of disaster, as specified in the policy. Homeowners' insurance applications may include a question about smoking. One insurer's application asks: "Is there a smoker in the household?" Because smokers in the household increase the danger of house fires, a discount is often available for households in which no one smokes.

An automobile insurance policy is a package containing various types of coverage that can be tailored to fit the applicant's needs. Policies can provide money for medical bills, property damage, and lost wages of third parties that result from a collision with the insured's vehicle where the insured was at fault. They can provide money to repair the insured's vehicle after a collision, or the cash value of the vehicle if it is "totaled," or pay for damage to the insured's vehicle in the event of theft, fire, vandalism, or natural disaster. They also can pay medical expenses of the insured and any passengers injured in a crash caused by the insured's vehicle. Most states require drivers to purchase specified types and amounts of automobile insurance coverage. Some insurers offer a discount to nonsmokers because drivers who don't smoke are less likely to be involved in motor vehicle crashes than drivers who do.

186 Smokers become disabled earlier and die younger than nonsmokers, often leaving their families to struggle financially.

On average, smokers suffer disabilities earlier in life and die sooner than nonsmokers. When the smoker is the breadwinner, his or her early disability or death can severely impact the family's finances. Even when the smoker has disability income insurance, this insurance pays only part of the amount the person was earning before the disability, and ordinarily pays nothing beyond age 65. Smoking-related disabilities may last for decades and entail medical expenses, part of which won't be covered by health insurance. If life insurance is inadequate, the early death of a breadwinner can leave a family in dire financial straits.

Take the case of a 45-year-old corporate manager who has smoked a pack and a half of cigarettes every day since he was 14 years old. He has a wife and three children, 18, 14, and 12. He has had a cigarette cough for years, but when he begins losing weight and coughing up blood, he sees a physician who diagnoses lung cancer. Chemotherapy and radiation treatments begin and he becomes too ill to work. His disability income benefits are 60 percent of his former salary. His 18-year-old son, who had planned to go to college, instead takes a minimum-wage job to help out. His wife, who has no job experience, finds a job as a cashier in a restaurant. The younger children must do some of the housework and nursing care. Three years after his diagnosis, the husband and father dies, leaving only a small amount of life insurance. The couple's plans to finish paying off their mortgage, put the children through college, and save for retirement during the last 20 years of the husband's working life—the years when he would have earned the highest income—have all gone up in smoke.

The early disability or death of a homemaker who cares for young children likewise impacts the family financially. Her (or his) services will have to be replaced somehow. The working spouse will have to pay for childcare and house-keeping, if he or she can afford it. If not, that spouse must be breadwinner, mother and father, housekeeper, and cook.

Everyone should try to have adequate health, disability income, and life insurance, but smokers have a special obligation to do this—and such insurance is usually more expensive for smokers than for nonsmokers. Millions of families have struggled financially because smoking caused a family member's early disability or death. In extreme cases where dependent children are left impoverished by the smoker's disability or death, welfare may be the only recourse.

187 **If you smoke, you may spend considerable amounts of money in an attempt to keep your hair, clothing, and home from smelling of tobacco smoke.**

If you smoke, you may fight a continuous battle against smelling of stale tobacco smoke. To get rid of odors, you may have to shampoo your hair and launder your clothes frequently. Smoke odors are stubborn. You may need to buy special laundry products designed to remove smoke odors when regular laundry detergent doesn't do the job. Clothes may have to be washed more than once to eliminate smoke odors. Clothes that are frequently washed wear out sooner.

For clothes that must be dry cleaned, some cleaners offer a process called ozone treatment to remove smoke odors. Ozone treatment costs considerably more than regular dry cleaning. And, of course, odor successfully removed returns the next time that you light up while wearing the clothing.

If you smoke indoors, tobacco smoke coats and permeates everything in your house. You may become accustomed to the odor of tobacco smoke, but someone who is unaccustomed will notice it immediately. To combat tobacco smoke odors, carpets, drapes, furniture, walls, windows, and pictures must be cleaned often. This cleaning can be expensive and wears out furnishings, which must then be replaced. Walls that are scrubbed frequently to remove tobacco smoke residue will have to be repainted more often. Therefore, you could save a good deal of money if no one smokes inside your house.

188 **Smoking can result in cigarette burns in your clothing, household furnishings, and automobile upholstery. Repairing these items can be costly.**

Smokers often spend considerable money repairing or replacing items with cigarette burns. Clothing is especially apt to get scorched or burned. Inexpensive items are usually replaced. A burn hole in an expensive suit or coat might be rewoven, but this is costly. One hundred dollars to reweave a burn hole is not unusual.

Upholstered furniture in smokers' homes is especially likely to get burn holes from live ashes or contact with a burning cigarette. Reupholstering a large piece of furniture can cost hundreds of dollars. Burns in carpets and automobile upholstery also can be costly to repair.

If a smoker forgets a lighted cigarette on the edge of a wooden table, desk, or chest, the surface will probably sustain a burn. Inexpensive wooden furniture might be repaired by the homeowner. However, expensive furniture usually must be repaired by a professional. Cigarette burns on laminate (Formica-type) countertops may require replacement of the laminate. One expert says that there is no good way to repair laminate.

You can avoid costly damage to your household furnishings by not smoking in your home. This also protects other members of the household from breathing secondhand smoke, a more important consideration.

189 If your house or automobile smells of stale tobacco smoke it may be difficult to sell, and will usually sell for less.

Real estate agents say that fresh-smelling houses sell more quickly and for more money. Bad smells can discourage potential buyers, even if the buyers like the house otherwise. One of the biggest culprits is the smell of stale tobacco smoke. Often, the owner is not even aware that his house smells of tobacco smoke, but if people have been smoking in the house for a long time, furniture, carpets, drapes, curtains, wallpaper, and even wallboard may be saturated with smoke. Removing the smell is likely to be difficult and expensive, and potential buyers know this. Professional smoke-residue cleaners may charge over $10,000 to deodorize a large house. And cleaners cannot guarantee that they can remove all smoke residue, especially in ventilation ducts.

Automobiles that smell of stale tobacco smoke present a similar problem. Because millions of people wouldn't consider buying an automobile in which someone has smoked, such automobiles are worth less on the used car market. Automobiles in which no one has smoked are often advertised as "nonsmoker," a positive selling point.

Some smokers think that their car won't smell if they open the windows while smoking, but this doesn't work. Over time, the upholstery and other interior surfaces become saturated with stale tobacco smoke whether the windows are open or not. Thus, in addition to the health and safety reasons not to smoke in houses and automobiles, there are economic reasons as well.

Costs to the Smoker's Career

190 **Employees who smoke cost employers more than employees who don't. For this and other reasons, smokers make less desirable employees and earn less, on average, than nonsmokers.**

Employers have become increasingly aware that employees who smoke cost them more than those who don't. Smokers use more sick time than nonsmokers, costing the employer in lost productivity, or in overtime pay to workers replacing them. A smoker is also more likely to become disabled or die than a nonsmoker. The employer then has to hire and train a replacement. The loss of even one key employee to smoking-related disability or death can hamper the employer's operations.

Many employers provide their employees with group health insurance. Smoking-related illnesses increase the cost of group health insurance and, in some cases, the employer absorbs the entire amount. If employees pay part or all of the premiums, the nonsmokers may pay the same amount as the smokers. If the nonsmokers feel that the smokers are costing them money, this can lower employee morale. To avoid this problem, some employers make smokers pay extra for their health insurance. Employees who smoke may also increase the employer's cost of group life and disability income insurance, unemployment insurance, and workers' compensation insurance.

Today, most employers ban smoking in the workplace or restrict it to specified areas. Employers that do not ban or restrict smoking put themselves at risk of costly lawsuits brought by employees claiming damage to their health from secondhand smoke. Allowing smoking in the workplace also increases cleaning costs and the likelihood of fire and injuries. Moreover, secondhand smoke can harm a company's computer hard drives. An employer has a legal right to ban or restrict smoking, unless the employer has entered into a union agreement to the contrary. Some state and local laws require employers to ban or restrict smoking.

While state laws may entitle employees to breaks during the workday, many employees who smoke take extra breaks to satisfy their nicotine cravings. Whether they smoke on the job or outdoors, these extra breaks make smokers less productive. One study of employees at an oil refinery found that smokers took smoke breaks totaling an hour and 36 minutes per 12-hour shift. A survey in Michigan found that the average employee who smokes takes three smoke breaks each workday. These breaks average 13 minutes each, or 39 minutes a workday.

If you smoke you may have difficulty getting hired. Many employers will count smoking against a job applicant. One company requires job applicants to pass a nicotine test. A bias against smokers also can occur when employees are being considered for promotion. Some employers do spot checks for nicotine and fire employees who smoke. One company executive said "We're not telling you you can't smoke. We're telling you you can't smoke and work here." Because they are less desirable employees, and have generally poorer health, smokers earn on average four to eight percent less than nonsmokers, even after taking into account education and experience.

191 Smoking is incompatible with many careers and professions.

For a variety of reasons, smoking is incompatible with certain careers and professions. Someone who aspires to be a professional ice skater, for instance, is unlikely to have the stamina to perform rigorous routines on the ice if he or she smokes. Other professional athletes, including football, basketball, baseball, and hockey players, must also avoid smoking in order to have the stamina to play well.

People in other professions that require high levels of physical fitness, or place stress on the lungs or heart, must not smoke. Included in this category are professional divers and mountain climbers, jet fighter pilots, and astronauts. Smoking is also incompatible with jobs that expose workers to radon, smoke, gases, or dusts, such as mining, firefighting, and many industrial occupations. Smoking, in addition to inhaling dangerous substances on the job, is playing Russian roulette with your health.

Many people in the entertainment industry must avoid smoking if they are to succeed. Professional dancers need strength and energy to perform, and smoking saps both. Professional horn and bagpipe players need large lung volume, a strong diaphragm, and good breath control, qualities likely to be lacking in smokers. The same is true of professional singers. Moreover, singers use their vocal cords as their instrument and smoking causes problems with the vocal cords, such as laryngitis and hoarseness. Colds and respiratory infections, more common in smokers, also interfere with a professional singer's ability to perform. For others in the entertainment industry, including radio and television announcers, talk show hosts, and stand-up comedians, a cigarette cough can end a career.

A cigarette cough will also be detrimental to the careers of people who appear before groups, including public speakers and teachers. Moreover, school boards and parents may view teachers who smoke as poor role models for young people. Many schools have antismoking programs for their students, beginning in kindergarten and continuing through high school. A teacher who smokes has the potential to undermine the school's efforts at smoking prevention.

People who work in the health professions—doctors, nurses, physical therapists, dentists, and dental hygienists—may lose credibility with patients if they smoke. Patients may wonder how a well-informed health professional could endanger his or her health by smoking, and will probably have less respect for that person's judgment. Also, health professionals often work in close physical proximity to their patients, and the smell of tobacco smoke on their hair, clothing, and breath is offensive to many patients.

Salespersons need to make a good impression on clients. If the salesperson is puffing on a cigarette, or smells of tobacco smoke, he or she may lose the sale. One real estate agent says, "I never smoke around my clients. They're actually prejudiced against smokers, so I never let them know." But "never letting them know" could be impossible if the salesperson smells of tobacco smoke.

192 Smokers, on average, recoup less from Social Security and Medicare than nonsmokers.

During their working years, smokers and nonsmokers pay at the same rate into the Social Security system, which includes Medicare. For the year 2009, the payroll tax rate for Social Security (FICA) was 6.20 percent of the employee's earnings, up to $106,800. The Medicare payroll tax rate was 1.45 percent, paid on all earnings. Because smokers on average die younger than nonsmokers, they recoup less of their payroll taxes from Social Security and Medicare.

For people born in 1938 and later, full Social Security benefits begin after age 65 (although a reduced benefit can be chosen as early as age 62). For example, people born in 1938 must wait until age 65 and 2 months, people born in 1939 must wait until age 65 and 4 months, and so forth. People born in 1960 and later must wait until age 67 to receive full benefits. Medicare services do not begin until age 65, except for some people with disabilities. Although smokers pay into the Social Security system at the same rates as nonsmokers, on average they receive benefits for fewer years than nonsmokers, and have a briefer period of eligibility for Medicare. Therefore, in the United States, smokers subsidize nonsmokers' retirements.

193 College graduates on average make more money than people who do not have a college education. High school students who smoke are less likely to earn merit or athletic scholarships that might enable them to go to college.

Many studies show that college graduates on average make more money than people who do not have a college education. Although most parents think a college education is important for their child, many can't finance that education. One study indicated that only seven percent of parents had saved enough to send their child to college, while 48 percent had saved from one to 50 percent of the cost. College costs vary widely. In 2008, yearly tuition, fees, and room and board cost $10,812 for in-state students at Western State College of Colorado, while a year at Sarah Lawrence College in New York cost $50,810. But even the lower-cost colleges may be out of reach for many who would like to attend college.

Often, loans, jobs, and scholarships have to make up the deficit. Merit or athletic scholarships offer a way to pay for part or all of college for thousands of students. Merit scholarships are based on academic achievement. Studies have shown that smokers on average get lower grades in high school than nonsmokers. The reason for this is unknown, but smoking and lower grades are unquestionably linked. Thus, high school students who smoke are less likely to earn merit scholarships.

The competition for athletic scholarships is intense, and a smoker is unlikely to make the grade. One qualification is a record of athletic success in high school, but most high school coaches don't want smokers on their teams. Coaches' careers depend on the success of the athletes they coach. Coaches know that smokers don't have the energy, endurance, and strength that athletes need. Moreover, even if a smoker is allowed to participate in high school sports, he or she is unlikely to perform well enough to earn an athletic scholarship.

Studies of smoking among young people have shown that African American teenagers are less likely to smoke than white teenagers. Researchers are uncertain about the reasons for this. But some African American students say they don't smoke because they view an athletic scholarship as their only route to higher education.

194 Some employers offer incentives to encourage employees not to smoke.

Some employers offer monetary or other incentives to encourage their employees not to smoke. At some companies, all nonsmoking employees pay less for group life and health insurance, are awarded extra time off, or given extra pay. Employers may subsidize smoking cessation programs. And in some states there are laws requiring employers to include smoking cessation treatment in their health insurance plans. When employees are successful in quitting, some employers offer money or other awards, typically an extra personal holiday or membership in a health club.

Smokers who do not have access to a subsidized smoking cessation program nevertheless have been befriended by the Internal Revenue Service (IRS). Under federal tax law, family medical expenses that exceed 7.5 percent of adjusted gross income are tax deductible. The IRS has ruled that smoking cessation programs and prescription drugs used to fight nicotine addiction are tax-deductible medical expenses.

Other Ways Smoking Costs Smokers

195 If you smoke, you may have difficulty renting living space. And your security deposit might be used for cleaning up, rather than returned to you. Even if you buy your own condominium, you might not be able to smoke there.

Landlords prefer to rent houses and apartments to non-smokers. Smoking increases the danger of fire. Landlords also fear complaints or lawsuits by tenants in adjoining apartments if tobacco smoke drifts into their living space. Moreover, smoking increases the difficulty of cleaning up when the smoker has vacated the apartment or house. In one extreme case, a landlord said that he had to replace the wallboard to get rid of the smell of tobacco smoke in an apartment where a tenant who smoked heavily had lived for ten years. In many cases, landlords have to use special paint on smoke-stained walls, and must replace burned carpeting and counters. One landlord said that on average it cost him $1,500 to clean a smoker's apartment, but only $400 to clean a nonsmoker's. Thus, if you smoke, your security deposit might be used for cleaning up, rather than returned to you.

Landlords have a legal right to ban smoking in rental property. Ads for rental units often specify "nonsmokers only," sometimes by the notation "N/S." The American Nonsmokers Rights Foundation suggests that the following language be included in apartment leases:

SMOKING: Due to the increased risk of fire, and the known health effects of secondhand smoke, smoking is prohibited in any area of the property, both private and common, whether enclosed or outdoors. This policy applies to all owners, tenants, guests, and servicepersons.

Similar language can be included in the governing documents of condominium complexes. Each apartment or townhouse in a condominium complex is separately owned, usually by the person who occupies it. But people who live in condominiums must abide by the rules that govern the entire complex. And, in 2008, a city in California passed an ordinance that bans smoking in any multistory, multi-dwelling building, either rental or condominium— perhaps a harbinger of things to come. So, even if you buy your own condominium, you may not be able to smoke there. Your home is not always your castle when you are a smoker.

196 Lawsuits against smokers who expose others to tobacco smoke have become increasingly common, and can be costly to smokers.

Apartment dwellers can be irritated or made ill by tobacco smoke drifting in from other places in the building. Increasingly, they have been complaining to landlords, condominium managers, and county health officials. Some complain that they have to open windows in the winter to air out their apartments, or close windows in the summer because neighbors are smoking on nearby balconies. Some say that smoke enters their apartments through ventilating systems. Action on Smoking and Health (ASH), the legal arm of the nonsmoking movement, has pointed out that, "Despite the best modern filtration systems, many of the carcinogenic and other dangerous components of tobacco smoke can be circulated through a building's circulation system."

In some cases, an aggrieved apartment dweller has sued the neighbor who smokes, the landlord, or both. The aggrieved apartment dweller (the plaintiff) can use one or more legal theories in the suit, including breach of the covenant of quiet enjoyment, nuisance, battery, trespass, intentional infliction of emotional distress, constructive eviction, and breach of the warranty of habitability. The plaintiffs have won most of these cases.

Employees have brought battery lawsuits against coworkers who exposed them to tobacco smoke. Battery means touching someone against his or her will, or putting in motion a substance that touches that person. A smoker is a fair target for a battery lawsuit if he or she continues to smoke around a person that the smoker knows has a special sensitivity to tobacco smoke, such as an allergy or asthma. In Georgia, an employee sued a coworker and the employer for battery, claiming that continual exposure to the coworker's pipe smoke made her sick. The Georgia court noted that tobacco smoke "is detectable through the senses and may be ingested or inhaled. It is capable of touching or making contact with one's person in a number of ways." Ordinarily, an employee who is made ill at work can be paid only through workers' compensation. However, if battery from contact with tobacco smoke can be established, the damages (money) that the defendant must pay can be much higher than workers' compensation payments.

A person has a legal right not to be touched in ways that are offensive and insulting to him or her. In Ohio, an antismoking activist was appearing as a guest on a radio program. The talk show host intentionally blew tobacco smoke in the activist's face. The activist sued, claiming "physical discomfort, humiliation, and distress." The Ohio appeals court held that a smoker could be liable for battery if he or she intentionally aims smoke at another person.

As people become more aware of the dangers of secondhand smoke, suits against smokers are increasingly common. A smoker who isn't careful to keep smoke away from other people could spend a considerable amount of money to defend such a suit. Moreover, the smoker is more likely than not to lose the suit. And a judgment against a smoker, especially a judgment allowing punitive damages (damages meant to punish the smoker), could be very costly.

197 If you are an underage smoker, or an adult who violates "no smoking" laws, you may be fined or otherwise punished.

States, cities, counties, and towns have a patchwork quilt of laws governing smoking. Some laws are aimed at employers or business owners, some at merchants who sell cigarettes, and others at smokers themselves. The number of laws governing smoking is growing rapidly. For example, in 1985 there were 175 communities with clean indoor air ordinances. Today, there are thousands.

Some states have statewide clean indoor air laws. Under Oregon's Smokefree Workplace Law, effective in 2002, with some exceptions, employers must post "No Smoking" signs and ensure that their workplaces are smoke-free. Violations can result in $1,000 fines for the employer in each 30-day period. An Oregon employer has little choice but to reprimand, and possibly fire, an employee who continues smoking in violation of the law.

Nevada's clean indoor air law, enacted in 2006, is aimed at smokers themselves. In Nevada it is a misdemeanor to smoke in many indoor places of employment. In addition to any criminal penalty, there is a civil penalty of $100. But the law does not apply to gaming areas of casinos.

Laws in an increasing number of states and communities prohibit smoking in restaurants. The purpose of these laws is to protect the health of restaurant workers and customers. For example, Maine imposes $100 fines on restaurant owners and customers who violate its restaurant smoking ban.

California, which prohibits smoking in bars as well as in restaurants, may impose fines of up to $7,000 on repeat violators of its law. The town of Hayward, California fines smokers $50 if they are caught smoking on sidewalks, streets, parks, sports fields, playgrounds, municipal parking lots, or no-smoking zones around outdoor patios of restaurants and bars.

A few laws provide sanctions for people smoking at home. Under a Massachusetts law, police officers and firefighters can be fired from their jobs if they smoke anywhere, including their own homes. The rationale is that state taxpayers have to pay disability costs when police officers and firefighters contract smoking-related illnesses. The Massachusetts Supreme Judicial Court has upheld this law.

In Montgomery County, Maryland, a person whose tobacco smoke wafts from his home into a neighbor's can be fined if he fails to take steps to solve the problem. The fines range up to $750 per violation.

In California, fines are levied against a person who throws a lighted cigarette from a motor vehicle. These fines range from $100 to $1,000, and an order to pick up litter or clean graffiti for a first conviction.

State laws prohibit merchants from selling tobacco to minors. Unfortunately, these laws are often laxly enforced. Moreover, studies show that even where these laws are enforced vigorously, young people are usually able to obtain cigarettes. New smokers may get them from friends who are over 18 or steal them from their parents. Some ask adult strangers to buy cigarettes for them or get them from cigarette vending machines. Teenage store clerks are a common source of cigarettes for high school students. Some young smokers shoplift cigarettes or use false identification to purchase them.

Because laws aimed at merchants are inadequate to prevent underage smoking, state and local governments are starting to pass laws aimed at the underage smokers themselves. In 1997, Florida passed a law forbidding people under 18 to buy, possess, or smoke tobacco. Special police forces, funded by money from a settlement with the tobacco industry, patrol malls and parks where teenagers hang out. Teenagers caught smoking must pay a fine of $53 or do eight hours of community service. A third violation results in automatic loss of the teenager's driver's license. A study showed that this law has cut down on teenage smoking by 40 percent.

An Ohio law that went into effect in 2001 makes it illegal for a person under 18 to buy, possess, or use tobacco or tobacco-related items, such as rolling paper. A juvenile judge can impose a fine of $100 or require the offender to attend tobacco use education classes. Failure to comply can result in an increased fine, 20 hours of community service, or a 30-day suspension of the offender's driver's license.

In California there is a law against a minor purchasing, receiving, or possessing tobacco products. It is also against California law to sell, give, or furnish tobacco products of any sort to people under age 18.

In Castle Rock, Colorado, an ordinance imposes a $300 fine on minors who smoke or possess tobacco products. Spokane County, in Washington State, has a similar law with a $95 fine. After this law was passed, in one week a Spokane County high school suspended 16 students who smoked on school grounds, which cut down considerably on smoking at this high school.

198 In order to purchase cigarettes, poor smokers often divert money from essentials.

Studies show that the poorer the smoker, the greater the proportion of income he or she is willing to spend on cigarettes. Thus, poor smokers often divert money from essentials to buy cigarettes. Teenage smokers may go without lunch to buy cigarettes. Old people living on pensions may go without food, medicines, clothing, or heat to buy cigarettes.

Even sadder are parents who deprive their children of essentials so that the parents can smoke. For example, Frank McCourt, in his Pulitzer-Prize-winning memoir, *Angela's Ashes*, described his poverty-stricken Irish childhood in which he and his siblings rarely had enough to eat, but his parents nevertheless bought cigarettes. McCourt says, "There may be a lack of tea or bread in the house but Mam and Dad always manage to get the fags, the Wild Woodbines. They have to have the Woodbines in the morning and anytime they drink tea."

Whenever federal or state governments consider raising cigarette taxes, the thorny problem of additional burdens on poor smokers must be confronted. On the one hand, more expensive cigarettes keep some young people from taking up smoking, and cause some smokers to quit. On the other hand, poor smokers may buy cigarettes that they and their families can ill afford.

Costs of Smoking to the Public

199 Fires ignited by smoking materials result in enormous monetary losses. Smokers and nonsmokers alike bear the costs of smoking-related fires.

Smoking-related fires are extremely costly. Smoking materials ignite fires that destroy houses, apartments, businesses, industrial facilities, public buildings, vehicles, timber, and crops. In 2005, these fires cause an estimated $575 million in property loss in the United States.

Smoking-related fires also result in enormous costs to treat fire victims. Burn centers have become more and more successful in saving the lives of burn victims. Although this is highly desirable, it also means that burn treatment has gotten much more costly. Treatment of a person with massive burns can cost hundreds of thousands of dollars. Treatment of a severe smoke inhalation injury usually means an expensive stay in a hospital intensive care unit or a burn center. Medical and transportation costs for treating victims of fires ignited by smoking materials are estimated to be $160 million a year.

Every year in the United States, smoking-related fires cause thousands of deaths and injuries. People who die or are seriously injured in smoking-related fires stop working. Thus, the goods and services that they otherwise would have produced are lost. The value to the economy of these lost goods and services is estimated at more than a billion dollars a year.

Smoking-related fires increase firefighting costs in this country by an estimated $186 million a year. When smoking rates decline, as they have in California for example, the decrease in the number of fires allows firefighters to spend more time providing other essential services, such as rendering emergency medical aid, dealing with hazardous materials, and fire prevention.

200 Smoking in public buildings and other public facilities causes a huge increase in maintenance costs. Everyone pays, smokers as well as nonsmokers.

Maintenance costs skyrocket in public buildings where smoking is allowed. In the 1990s, U.S. government economists estimated that $4 billion to $8 billion a year could be saved through reduced maintenance if smoking were banned in all public buildings. Where smoking is banned, furniture and drapes last longer and many cleaning chores can be done less often. Where smoking is allowed, the extra maintenance costs are passed on to the public. Everyone pays, smokers as well as nonsmokers.

Businesses that cater to the public may pass the costs of maintaining their facilities on to their customers. When such businesses ban smoking, their maintenance costs decrease markedly. One airline reported that it saved hundreds of thousands of dollars a year in maintenance costs after it banned smoking on its flights. A spokesperson for the airline said, "Smoke dirties air filters, carpets, seat covers. And then there's the man-hours required to empty ash trays after every flight."

Most hotels now set aside a majority of rooms for nonsmokers due to the large growth in requests for nonsmoking rooms. Nonsmokers don't like to stay in a hotel room that smells of stale tobacco smoke. When hotel housekeepers find evidence that a guest has smoked in a nonsmoking room, hotels have elaborate (and expensive) procedures to clean the room. They dry clean draperies and bedspreads, launder sheer curtains, shampoo the carpet, change filters on the heating and air-conditioning system, and clean the furniture and fixtures. These costs may be passed on to all customers in the form of higher prices. But one hotel charges any guest who smokes in its rooms a $250 cleaning fee—the amount hotel management says it costs to get rid of the smell of tobacco smoke.

201 **Millions of cigarette butts are disposed of improperly every year, increasing unsightly litter and making costly cleanup necessary. If you smoke, be careful where you dispose of cigarette litter. Smokers pay for cleanup, along with everyone else.**

Smoking is banned in more and more workplaces and public buildings, so more people go outside to smoke, increasing cigarette litter on streets and sidewalks, especially where there is a lack of ashtrays and trash receptacles. Moreover, in the 1990s, car manufacturers began to make ashtrays an option that adds to the price of the car. Some smokers throw cigarette butts out of their car windows because they are driving a car that has no ashtrays.

Littering on highways, streets, sidewalks, parks, and beaches is a problem everywhere. Cigarette butts are the most littered item, both in this country and abroad. Every year in the United States, millions of cigarette butts are disposed of improperly. On International Coastal Cleanup Day, which is held in September of each year, between one and two million cigarette butts, cigar tips, tobacco wrappers, and cigarette lighters are removed from ocean, lake, and river beaches in the United States. Cigarette filters are made of a plastic called cellulose acetate that can take up to five years to break down. So a cigarette butt that is not removed from the landscape remains an eyesore for years. One woman said, "I will never understand why some people who smoke cigarettes think the world is their personal ashtray."

Cleaning up cigarette litter is expensive. Paid workers remove much of it. For example, Pennsylvania State University officials say that it costs $150,000 a year for maintenance crews to clean up campus cigarette litter.

Volunteers clean up a lot of litter, but that doesn't mean it's entirely free. It costs money to recruit and equip volunteers, and to transport litter to a landfill. Offenders—prisoners, probationers, and parolees—also clean up some litter but, again, their work is not free. Paid overseers must accompany offenders. Offenders have to be equipped, transported, and fed, all of which costs money.

And discarded cigarette butts that haven't been extinguished are hazardous. A smoldering cigarette butt lying on a beach could cause a painful burn if someone with bare feet stepped on it. Wildland fires have been started when a lighted cigarette butt was thrown out of a car window. Buildings have burned down when someone who thought the cigarette was extinguished tossed it into a wastebasket. In 2009, newpapers reported that a bird building a nest in the eave of a building was lining the nest with discarded cigarette butts, one of which was still lighted. The nest and then the roof of the building caught fire, resulting in nearly half a million dollars in damage. So if you smoke, be careful how you dispose of cigarette butts. Better yet, quit smoking for all the reasons discussed in this book.

HELPING OTHERS QUIT TOBACCO

In *Smoking: 201 Reasons to Quit,* I have primarily addressed the tobacco user, citing everything from the increased risks of disease to increased insurance premiums. As I say in the Afterword, I hope these reasons will persuade those who don't smoke to refuse to even consider using tobacco, and those who smoke to quit. But I have only peripherally addressed the role of third parties in persuading someone who hasn't started not to start, or helping a smoker to quit.

People quit any bad habit only when they are motivated to quit. Giving a family member, friend, or significant other a copy of *Smoking: 201 Reasons to Quit* is a good beginning. Be sure that the smoker knows that you are giving him the book out of concern for him. And read the book yourself, even if you think that's preaching to the choir. This will help you find specific reasons to quit that may be convincing to a smoker you know well. For instance, if your husband has remained unpersuaded for 20 years, as the health dangers of smoking have become ever more alarming, you already know that no amount of evidence is going to get him to quit for his own health. But you may be able to appeal to that nagging concern he has about the effects of secondhand smoke on your children. Or about the example his smoking is setting them. Or maybe he cannot figure out why he is repeatedly passed over for promotion when his work is highly regarded by bosses and coworkers.

If you have a close friend who insists that there's no point in quitting because the damage has already been done, you can point out to her that her risk for some diseases and disabilities begins to reverse almost immediately after quitting, and other risks decline when she remains smoke-free for a number of years. You may be able to persuade her that its never too late to quit.

If you are trying to convince a teenager to quit—or not to start in the first place—you have probably already stumbled over the I-don't-care-about-all-those-dumb-diseases-that-old-people-get roadblock. Concentrate instead on countering the image promoted by the tobacco industry that smoking makes you appear popular, sophisticated, or "cool." When teenagers learn that smokers have bad breath, develop wrinkles, and lose their teeth and hair at younger ages, and that nonsmokers don't want to date smokers, much less marry them, they are less apt to see smoking as glamorous. And learning that their scholarship opportunities can be decreased by tobacco use is more likely to impress a teenager than the threat of disease.

Never nag a smoker about their smoking—it's likely to be counterproductive. But be as persistent as you can without alienating the smoker. If both you and your sister smoke, suggest to her that you quit together. Offer your mother moral support and breakfast in bed every day during the time she is quitting. Tell your spouse that the two of you can take a long-deferred dream vacation with the money saved by not smoking. Some parents have successfully kept their children from using tobacco with the promise of a car at graduation, or a paid college education. Almost any device you can think of is worth a try. Such efforts may be more successful if you wait for the smoker to bring up the subject. A conversation such as the following probably would not alienate a smoker:

"I know I should quit smoking. I can't breathe anymore. But I just can't give it up."

"Well, is there a way I can help you? Maybe we can go to a spa where smoking isn't allowed. We've been through a lot together. We can get through this, too. I want you around for a long time."

If you are close to someone who has made numerous efforts to quit, but hasn't yet succeeded, reassure him that it's not hopeless, that most smokers make several attempts before they are successful and that there are new resources available to assist him in quitting. Be prepared to help. And tell him how proud you are that he is making the effort to quit.

Find out from the smoker what support he needs while he is quitting. Different people need different types of support. Once your smoker has quit, celebrate his success and continue to give him your support. There are many ways you can do this. If he suggests going to a smoky bar, offer to provide drinks at home instead. If smoking is allowed in his workplace, support him in his efforts to find a smoke-free workplace. Be available if he needs help against relapse. And if he relapses, remind him again that it usually takes smokers several tries before they are successful in quitting permanently. Your efforts are extremely important—literally a matter of life and death.

AFTERWORD

My involvement with smoking began in early childhood. My father smoked heavily. During his waking hours, I never saw him without a cigarette in his hand. I could tell where he was in the house by listening for his constant cough. His smoking upset my mother, a nonsmoker. I always felt my father's smoking was a factor that led to my parents' divorce, which occurred when I was 15.

When I was an adult, my father was diagnosed with emphysema, a lung disease nearly always caused by smoking. Then he suffered a stroke that left him partially paralyzed. He spent years going between his bed and a motorized wheelchair. He was hooked up to an oxygen tank, but even so he could not comfortably walk across the room. He quit smoking only when the people who managed his nursing home took away his cigarettes, fearing that the combination of oxygen and smoking would cause a fire. At one point, my father tried to drive his motorized wheelchair down a highway from the nursing home to a grocery store—undoubtedly intending to buy cigarettes! When I was in law school he died of a heart attack.

After law school, I worked as a lawyer for a life and health insurance company. For many years, my duties included studying hundreds of medical files relating to insurance claims, and conferring with physicians who also worked for the company. In the course of studying these files, I took note of how many illnesses were caused or made worse by tobacco use.

Later, I made an independent study of the effects of tobacco. I learned that there are more than 60,000 medical journal articles about tobacco's harmful impact on health, and thousands of magazine and newspaper articles about tobacco's adverse effects on personal, social, and legal relationships, on physical appearance, and on financial well-being.

Although a great deal has been written about tobacco use in medical journals, magazines, and newspapers, little appears on the shelves of bookstores and libraries. In many bookstores, there are hundreds of books about diet and exercise, but few or none specifically about the hazards of tobacco use. Yet tobacco use is as great a health hazard as a poor diet or lack of exercise. Clearly, there is a need for a book with a comprehensive look at the hazards of tobacco use.

While my father is a prime example of the hazards of tobacco use, my brother is a prime example of the benefits of quitting smoking. Following my father's example, my brother began smoking at age 14. But, unlike my father, my brother was a light smoker and quit smoking at age 34. He is now the age that my father was when he died. When I called to talk to my brother the other day, his wife said, "He's out jogging." How much better to be out jogging than to be dying because you didn't quit smoking!

I would be delighted to hear from readers, especially those who have struggled with an addiction to tobacco, or who are distressed by the smoking of a family member or friend. You can write to me in care of Dillon & Parker Publishing LLC, P.O. Box 504, Walnut Creek, CA 94597-0504.

Persuasion has been a big part of my job as a lawyer. I hope that through this book I can persuade some people not to begin using tobacco and others to quit. No persuasion I have ever done could be as important as that.

Muriel L. Crawford

DEDICATION

This book is dedicated to my family members, friends, and acquaintances who have quit smoking. They are: John Henderson; Sharon Taylor; Bill Hall; Frank and John Des Ilets; Ralph Robinson; Jean Raymond; Mary, Ted, and Scott Schwartz; William Snyder; Susan and Bob Shaw; Arnold and Robert Taylor; Dustyn Deakins; Dorothy Scarlett; Susan Charles; Jim and Joanne Kidd; Sam and Jon Spieler; Dorothy Wurlitzer; Tony and Linda Tirdel; Vivien Warren; Karen Kushner; Igor Kipnis; Dietlind Goricke; Tom Bacon; Dan Payne; E. J. Simpson; Robert Walley, D.D.S.; Anna Mirtseva; Shirley and Louis Rauscher; Jim Ruegg; Gayle Buxton; Lisa Kozlowski; Lisa Meyers; Elaine Welch; Valerie Wolf; Julie Wolley; Sheree Murray; Laura Kelly; Hector Juan Brane; James Brooks; Gigi Loughner; Sheila Santini; Charles Barlow; Cynthia Brumley; Debby Hull; Sarah Scott-Farber; Jack and Pat O'Donnell; Tom and Deb Kelly; Larry Convento; Karen and Jack Friedman; and Brian Kolberg.

ACKNOWLEDGMENTS

Many people have helped to produce this book. My daughter, Barbara E. Crawford, M.L.I.S., who is expert in information technology and computers, helped with the research and solved technical problems. My husband, Barrett Crawford, edited the manuscript. Registered nurses Janet M. Crawford (also my daughter), David A. Taylor, Andrea Tran, and Linda Tirdel read portions or all of the manuscript and provided many useful suggestions.

I am grateful to the eminent members of the Medical Advisory Panel, who provided guidance and assured that the medical information in this book is correct. I also want to thank other physicians and dentists who read and commented on sections of the book related to their specialties: Jeffrey T. Bortz, M.D., Michael I. Turan, M.D., Alfred M. Peretti, M.D., Krishan Goel, M.D., Kevin S. Adair, D.D.S., and Robert Walley, D.D.S. The material about gene damage was review by Professor of Genetics Dean Robinson, Ph.D. Fire Captain Tom Mota commented on the material about fires. Gilbert Byers, M.D., read the entire manuscript.

Finally, this book would never have been published without the help of book shepard Alan Gadney and book designer Carolyn Porter of One-On-One Book Production and Marketing. Their decades-long experience was invaluable. And my thanks to Peri Poloni-Gabriel, of Knockout Design, who created the eye-catching book cover.

My sincere gratitude to all those who have helped me.

MEDICAL ADVISORY PANEL

Alex A. Adjei, M.D., Ph. D.—Practice in oncology. Senior Vice President of Clinical Research, Chairman, Department of Medicine, and the Katherine Anne Gioia Chair in Cancer Medicine, Roswell Park Cancer Institute. Dr. Adjei speaks and publishes extensively in his medical specialties—lung cancer and the development of novel drugs for cancer treatment. Recipient of numerous international awards and research grants. Member of the American Society for Clinical Pharmacology and Therapeutics; International Society for the Study of Lung Cancer; American Association for Cancer Research; American Society of Clinical Oncology; American Association for the Advancement of Science; American College of Physicians; and Ghana Medical Association. Graduate, University of Ghana Medical School, Accra (1982). Doctorate in Pharmacology, University of Edmonton, Alberta (1989). Internships, residencies, and consultancies at Howard University, Johns Hopkins School of Medicine, and Mayo Clinic and Foundation. Board certified in internal medicine and oncology.

Andrew Bruce Barnett, M.D.—Practice in reconstructive and cosmetic surgery. Chief of Plastic Surgery at St. Francis Memorial Hospital, San Francisco. Past Chief of Staff, Bay Area Surgery Center. Expert's Panel, American Burn Association. Developed a dressing used extensively for burn and wound healing. Member, American Society for Aesthetic Plastic Surgery; American Society of Plastic Surgeons. Member of Interplast, an association of medical professionals who donate reconstructive surgery in Third World countries. Dr. Barnett publishes and lectures on subjects related to his specialty and has received awards for his work. Graduate of Johns Hopkins School of Medicine. Resident at Stanford University Medical Center. Board certified in plastic surgery.

Gerald S. Berenson, M.D.—Practice in cardiology. Research Professor of Medicine, Pediatrics, Biochemistry, and Epidemiology, Tulane Center for Cardiovascular Health; Director, Tulane Center for Cardiovascular Health; and Director of the Bogalusa Heart Study, Tulane University. Emeritus Boyd Professor, Louisiana State University Medical School. Recipient of many honors and awards, Dr. Berenson has authored four books and hundreds of articles and has served on the boards of several peer-reviewed journals. Served on numerous Councils of the American Heart Association. Past President of the Louisiana Heart Association (1971). Fellow of the American College of Physicians (1963-). Member of professional associations with specialties in hypertension, nutrition, preventive cardiology, cardiovascular diseases, and geriatric cardiology. Graduate of Tulane University Medical School (1945), with postgraduate work at U.S. Naval Hospital, Bethesda, Maryland; University of Chicago; Louisiana State University; and several other institutions. Board certified in internal medicine.

Arnold R. Brody, Ph.D.—Research scientist in respiratory disease, educator. Professor and Vice Chairman, Department of Pathology, School of Medicine, Tulane University Health Sciences Center, New Orleans. Laboratory Director, National Institute of Environmental Health Sciences Research, Triangle Park, North Carolina (1978-93). Dr. Brody has authored more than 40 chapters in books and 115 articles in professional journals. Member of the editorial boards of pathology and toxicology journals. Recipient of numerous research grants from the National

Institutes of Health. Ph.D., Colorado State University (1969); Postdoctoral Fellow, Ohio State University (1969-72).

Michael L. Cohen, M.D.—Practice in pulmonology. Medical Director, Contra Costa Sleep Center, Walnut Creek, California. Medicare Medical Advisor Consultant. Director, National Association of Medical Directors of Respiratory Care. Past Chairman, John Muir Medical Center Department of Medicine. Past President, Alameda/ Contra Costa Medical Association. American Medical Association Delegate. Numerous other past professional activities, including professorships, directorships, chairmanships, consultancies. Graduate, University of Cincinnati, College of Medicine (1963). Residencies, Boston City Hospital and Boston Veteran's Administration Hospital. Intensive residency in occupational medicine, University of California at San Francisco (1984). Board certified in internal medicine, pulmonary disease, and sleep medicine.

Myles P. Cunningham, M.D.—Practice in medical oncology. Past president, American Cancer Society. Graduate, Feinberg School of Medicine, Northwestern University, Evanston, Illinois (1958). Residencies, Memorial Sloan-Kettering Cancer Center, New York; Columbus-Cuneo-Cabrini Medical Center and Cook County Hospital, Chicago. Board certified in surgery.

Lee R. Duffner, M.D., F.A.C.S.—Practice in ophthalmology. Emeritus Director, American Board of Ophthalmology (Director 1995-2002). Editor, *EyeNet,* Journal of the American Academy of Opthalmology. Maintenance of Certification Self-Assessment Reviewer, American Academy of Ophthalmology. Graduate, Medical College of Wisconsin, Milwaukee (1962). Residencies, University of Miami/ Jackson Memorial Medical Center and Stanford University Hospital, Palo Alto, California. Board certified in ophthalmology.

John H. Epstein, M.D.—Practice in dermatology. Clinical Professor of Dermatology, University of California at San Francisco School of Medicine. Past President, American Academy of Dermatology. Emeritus Director, American Board of Dermatology (Director 1974-1984). Past Vice President, Society of Investigative Dermatology. Marion B. Shulzberger International Lectureship (1985). Master in Dermatology, American Academy of Dermatology (1991). Clark W. Finnerud Award, Dermatology Foundation. Graduate, University of California at San Francisco School of Medicine (1952). Residencies, Mayo Graduate School of Medicine, Rochester, Minnesota, and Stanford University Hospital, Palo Alto, California. Board certified in dermatology.

Valentin Fuster, M.D., Ph.D.—Practice and research in cardiology. Past President of the American Heart Association. Immediate Past President of the World Heart Federation. Director of the Mount Sinai Cardiovascular Institute, New York. Richard Gorlin, M.D./Heart Research Foundation Professor of Cardiology, Mount Sinai School of Medicine. Dr. Fuster is the recipient of numerous grants and awards for research, holds honorary degrees from sixteen universities worldwide, and has authored, coauthored, or edited numerous books and more than 400 articles on coronary disease, atherosclerosis, and thrombosis. Editor-in-Chief of *Nature*; Clinical Practice Cardiovascular Medicine. Graduate, Faculty of Medicine, Barcelona University, Spain (1967). Internship in Medicine, Hospital Clinico, Barcelona; research fellowship, Edinburgh University, Scotland; residency in cardiology, Mayo Graduate School of Medicine, Rochester, Minnesota. Board certified in internal medicine and cardiovascular disease.

Earnestine Willis, M.D., M.P.H.—Practice in pediatrics. Associate Professor, Past Director of the Center for the Advancement of Urban Children, and Associate Dean of Multicultural Student Affairs, Medical College of Wisconsin, Milwaukee. Past Chair, Wisconsin Tobacco Control Board. Affiliated with many community organizations that promote the health of children and adolescents. Graduate of Harvard Medical School and Master's Degree at Harvard School of Public Health (1977). Residency and fellowship, Case Western Reserve University, Cleveland, Ohio. Fellowships, General Pediatrics, Leadership in Communities, Leadership Greater Chicago, Illinois, and Health Policy, Robert Wood Johnson University Hospital, New Brunswick, New Jersey. Board certified in pediatrics.

.

INDEX

cravings 110, 133, 161-162, 169, 170, 172, 173, 179, 229, 232, 268, 291
high blood pressure 16
increasing risk of low-birth-weight baby 130
increasing side effects of ergot and high blood pressure medications 148
inhibiting production of saliva 83
interaction with carbon monoxide 9, 22, 23-24
poisoning 8-9, 225-227
possible cause of hearing loss 91
possible cause of macular degeneration 88
preventing sleep 110
reducing the effectiveness of nitroglycerine 24
slowing healing of injured muscles and ligaments 98-99
slowing wound healing 105
triggering heart arrhythmias 28
withdrawal in newborns of mothers who smoke 132-133
working in opposition to angina medications 147
Nicotine Anonymous 174
Nitroglycerine
reduced effectiveness in smokers 24
to treat angina 24
Non-steroidal anti-inflammatory drugs (NSAIDS) causing peptic ulcer disease 83
to treat menstrual pain 116
Notobacco.org 174
NSAIDS (see Non-steroidal anti-inflammatory drugs)
Nursing home fires 207-208

NuvaRing 117

O

Obsessive-compulsive disorder 71
Occupational pollution 143-145
Occupational Safety and Health Administration 141, 210
Open chest surgery
to repair an aortic aneurysm 20
Oral contraceptives (See Birth control, pills)
Oregon's Smokefree Workplace Law 300
Organ transplants 18, 108, 152-153
waiting lists and smokers 152-153
Osteopenia 94
Osteoporosis 94-97
back pain from 98, 99
bone fractures from 95, 97, 98, 99
disability from 5
dowager's hump from 95, 244
earlier occurrence in women 94-95
falls 228-229
hormone replacement therapy 96,119
lupus 102
periodontal disease 76
protection from by diet 11, 95-96
risk of from smoking 96, 99, 102, 182, 228, 244
Outdoor air pollution 138-139
Outdoor barbeque grills
fire danger from smoking 217
Oxygen and
angina 23